FOOD SCIENCE AND TECHNOLOGY

# FOOD ALLERGY: OVERVIEW AND CHILDREN'S HEALTH ISSUES

## LEE R. DANIELS
### EDITOR

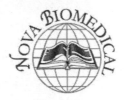

**Nova Science Publishers, Inc.**
*New York*

## NOTICE TO THE READER

LIBRARY OF CONGRESS CATALOGING-IN-PUBLICATION DATA

*Food allergy : overview and children's health issues / editor, Lee R. Daniels.*

*p. ; cm.*
*Includes index.*
*ISBN 978-1-61728-478-6 (hardcover)*
*1. Food allergy. 2. Food allergy--United States. 3. Food allergy in children. 4. Food allergy in children--United States. I. Daniels, Lee R.*
*[DNLM: 1. Food Hypersensitivity--United States. 2. Expert Testimony--United States. 3. Health Policy--United States. WD 310 F6862 2010]*
*RC596.F666 2010*
*618.92'975--dc22*

*2010022889*

Published by Nova Science Publishers, Inc. † New York

# FOOD ALLERGY: OVERVIEW AND CHILDREN'S HEALTH ISSUES

# FOOD SCIENCE AND TECHNOLOGY

Additional books in this series can be found on Nova's website under the Series tab.


Additional E-books in this series can be found on Nova's website under the E-book tab.

# CONTENTS

# PREFACE

Food allergy is an immunologic disease responsible for significant morbidity and is frequently accompanied by other allergic diseases including atopic dermatitis and asthma, and asthma is an important risk factor for severe allergic reactions to food. Patients with food allergy may have mild reactions, such as hives, but are also at risk for anaphylaxis, a severe and life-threatening systemic allergic reaction characterized by hives, fall of blood pressure, upper airway obstruction, and severe wheezing. This book explores food allergies which has emerged as an important public health problem based on its increasing prevalance, persistence throughout life, and potential for fatal reactions.

Chapter 1 - Food allergy affects up to 6 to 8 percent of children under the age of 3 and close to 4 percent of adults. If you have an unpleasant reaction to something you have eaten, you might wonder if you have a food allergy. One out of three people either believe they have a food allergy or modify their or their family's diet. Thus, while food allergy is commonly suspected, healthcare providers diagnose it less frequently than most people believe.

This pamphlet describes allergic reactions to foods and their possible causes as well as the best ways to diagnose and treat allergic reactions to food. It also describes other reactions to foods, known as food intolerances, which can be confused with food allergy, and describes some unproven and controversial food allergy theories.

Chapter 2 - Food allergies can range from merely irritating to life-threatening. Approximately 30,000 Americans go to the emergency room each year to get treated for severe food allergies, according to the Food Allergy and Anaphylaxis Network (FAAN). It is estimated that 150 to 200 Americans die each year because of allergic reactions to food.

Chapter 3 - Food allergy is a potentially serious immune response to eating specific foods or food additives. Eight types of food account for over 90% of allergic reactions in affected individuals: milk, eggs, peanuts, tree nuts, fish, shellfish, soy, and wheat [1,2]. Reactions to these foods by an allergic person can range from a tingling sensation around the mouth and lips and hives to death, depending on the severity of the allergy. The mechanisms by which a person develops an allergy to specific foods are largely unknown. Food allergy is more prevalent in children than adults, and a majority of affected children will "outgrow" food allergies with age. However, food allergy can sometimes become a lifelong concern [1]. Food allergies can greatly affect children and their families' well-being. There are some indications that the prevalence of food allergy may be increasing in the United States and in other countries [2–4].

Chapter 4 - Each year, millions of Americans have allergic reactions to food. Although most food allergies cause relatively mild and minor symptoms, some food allergies can cause severe reactions, and may even be life-threatening.

There is no cure for food allergies. Strict avoidance of food allergens — and early recognition and management of allergic reactions to food — are important measures to prevent serious health consequences.

Chapter 5 - The Food Allergen and Consumer Protection Act of 2004 (Public Law 108-282) requires the Secretary of Health and Human Services, acting through the Director of the National Institutes of Health (NIH), to convene an *ad hoc* panel of experts in allergy and immunology to review current basic and clinical research efforts related to food allergies, and requires that the panel make recommendations to the Secretary for enhancing and coordinating research activities concerning food allergies.

Chapters 6 through 10 feature testimony before the U. S. Senate.

In: Food Allergy Overview and Children's...      ISBN: 978-1-61728-478-6
Editor: Lee R. Daniels                    © 2010 Nova Science Publishers, Inc.

*Chapter 1*

# FOOD ALLERGY: AN OVERVIEW*

## *U.S. Department of Health and Human Services*

### INTRODUCTION

Food allergy affects up to 6 to 8 percent of children under the age of 3 and close to 4 percent of adults. If you have an unpleasant reaction to something you have eaten, you might wonder if you have a food allergy. One out of three people either believe they have a food allergy or modify their or their family's diet. Thus, while food allergy is commonly suspected, healthcare providers diagnose it less frequently than most people believe.

This pamphlet describes allergic reactions to foods and their possible causes as well as the best ways to diagnose and treat allergic reactions to food. It also describes other reactions to foods, known as food intolerances, which can be confused with food allergy, and describes some unproven and controversial food allergy theories.

---

* This is an edited, reformatted and augmented version of a U. S. Department of Health and Human Services publication dated July 2007.

# WHAT IS FOOD ALLERGY?

Food allergy is an abnormal response to a food triggered by the body's **immune system**. In this pamphlet, food allergy refers to a particular type of response of the immune system in which the body produces what is called an allergic, or IgE, **antibody** to a food. (IgE, or **immunoglobulin** E, is a type of protein that works against a specific food.)

Allergic reactions to food can cause serious illness and, in some cases, death. Therefore, if you have a food allergy, it is extremely important for you to work with your healthcare provider to find out what food(s) causes your allergic reaction.

Sometimes, a reaction to food is not an allergy at all but another type of reaction called "food intolerance."

Food intolerance is more common than food allergy. The immune system does not cause the symptoms of food intolerance, though these symptoms may look and feel like those of a food allergy.

*Note: Words in **bold** are defined in the glossary at the end of this booklet.*

# HOW DO ALLERGIC REACTIONS WORK?

An immediate allergic reaction involves two actions of your immune system

- Your immune system produces IgE. This protein is called a food-specific antibody, and it circulates through your blood.
- The food-specific IgE then attaches to **mast cells** and **basophils**. Basophils are found in blood. Mast cells are found in body tissues, especially in areas of your body that are typical sites of allergic reactions. Those sites include your nose, throat, lungs, skin, and **gastrointestinal (GI) tract**.

Generally, your immune system will form IgE against a food if you come from a family in which allergies are common —not necessarily food allergies but perhaps other allergic diseases, such as hay fever or asthma. If you have two allergic parents, you are more likely to develop food allergy than someone with one allergic parent.

If your immune system is inclined to form IgE to certain foods, you must be exposed to the food before you can have an allergic reaction.

As this food is digested, it triggers certain cells in your body to produce a food-specific IgE in large amounts. The food-specific IgE is then released and attaches to the surfaces of mast cells and basophils.

- The next time you eat that food, it interacts with food-specific IgE on the surface of the mast cells and basophils and triggers those cells to release chemicals such as **histamine**.
- Depending on the tissue in which they are released, these chemicals will cause you to have various symptoms of food allergy.

---

## CROSS-REACTIVE FOOD ALLERGIES

If you have a life-threatening reaction to a certain food, your healthcare provider will show you how to avoid similar foods that might trigger this reaction. For example, if you have a history of allergy to shrimp, allergy testing will usually show that you are not only allergic to shrimp but also to crab, lobster, and crayfish. This is called "cross-reactivity."

Another interesting example of cross-reactivity occurs in people who are highly sensitive to ragweed. During ragweed pollen season, they sometimes find that when they try to eat melons, particularly cantaloupe, they experience itching in their mouths and simply cannot eat the melon. Similarly, people who have severe birch pollen allergy also may react to apple peels. This is called the "oral allergy syndrome."

---

Food **allergens** are proteins in the food that enter your bloodstream after the food is digested. From there, they go to target organs, such as your skin or nose, and cause allergic reactions.

An allergic reaction to food can take place within a few minutes to an hour. The process of eating and digesting food affects the timing and the location of a reaction.

- If you are allergic to a particular food, you may first feel itching in your mouth as you start to eat the food.
- After the food is digested in your stomach, you may have GI symptoms such as vomiting, diarrhea, or pain.

- When the food allergens enter and travel through your bloodstream, they may cause your blood pressure to drop.
- As the allergens reach your skin, they can cause hives or eczema.
- When the allergens reach your mouth and lungs, they may cause throat tightness and trouble breathing.

## COMMON FOOD ALLERGIES

In adults, the foods that most often cause allergic reactions include

- Shellfish such as shrimp, crayfish, lobster, and crab
- Peanuts
- Tree nuts such as walnuts
- Fish
- Eggs

The most common foods that cause problems in children are

- Eggs
- Milk
- Peanuts
- Tree nuts

Peanuts and tree nuts are the leading causes of the potentially deadly food allergy reaction called **anaphylaxis**.

Adults usually keep their allergies for life, but children sometimes outgrow them. Children are more likely to outgrow allergies to milk, egg, or soy, however, than allergies to peanuts. The foods to which adults or children usually react are those foods they eat often. In Japan, for example, rice allergy is frequent. In Scandinavia, codfish allergy is common.

## FOOD ALLERGY OR FOOD INTOLERANCE?

If you go to your healthcare provider and say, "I think I have a food allergy," your provider has to consider other possibilities that may cause symptoms and could be confused with food allergy, such as food intolerance.

To find out the difference between food allergy and food intolerance, your provider will go through a list of possible causes for your symptoms. This is called a "differential diagnosis." This type of diagnosis helps confirm that you do indeed have a food allergy rather than a food intolerance or other illness.

## Types of Food Intolerance

### Food poisoning

One possible cause of symptoms like those of food allergy is food contaminated with **microbes**, such as bacteria, and **bacterial** products, such as **toxins**. Contaminated meat and dairy products sometimes cause symptoms, including GI discomfort, that resemble a food allergy when it is really a type of food poisoning.

### Histamine toxicity

There are substances, such as the powerful chemical histamine, present in certain foods that cause a reaction similar to an allergic reaction. For example, histamine can reach high levels in cheese, some wines, and certain kinds of fish such as tuna and mackerel.

In fish, histamine is believed to come from contamination by bacteria, particularly in fish that are not refrigerated properly. If you eat one of these foods with a high level of histamine, you could have a reaction that strongly resembles an allergic reaction to food. This reaction is called "**histamine toxicity**."

### Lactose intolerance

Another cause of food intolerance confused with a food allergy is lactose intolerance or **lactase deficiency**. This common food intolerance affects at least 1 out of 10 people.

Lactase is an **enzyme** that is in the lining of your gut. Lactase breaks down or digests lactose, a sugar found in milk and most milk products.

Lactose intolerance, or lactase deficiency, happens when there is not enough lactase in your gut to digest lactose. In that case, bacteria in your gut use lactose to form gas which causes bloating, abdominal pain, and sometimes diarrhea.

Your healthcare provider can use laboratory tests to find out whether your body can digest lactose.

---

### *Food additives*

Another type of food intolerance is a reaction to certain products that are added to food to enhance taste, provide color, or protect against the growth of microbes. Several chemical compounds, such as MSG (monosodium glutamate) and sulfites, are tied to reactions that can be confused with food allergy.

### MSG

MSG is a flavor enhancer and, when taken in large amounts, can cause some of the following signs:

- Flushing
- Sensations of warmth
- Headache
- Chest discomfort
- Feelings of detachment

These passing reactions occur rapidly after eating large amounts of food to which MSG has been added.

### Sulfites

Sulfites occur naturally in foods or may be added to increase crispness or prevent mold growth.

Sulfites in high concentrations sometimes pose problems for people with severe asthma. Sulfites can give off a gas called sulfur dioxide that a person with asthma inhales while eating food containing sulfites. This gas irritates the lungs and can send an asthmatic into severe bronchospasm, a tightening of the lungs.

The Food and Drug Administration (FDA) has banned sulfites as spray-on preservatives in fresh fruits and vegetables. Sulfites are still used in some foods, however, and occur naturally during the fermentation of wine.

### *Gluten intolerance*

Gluten intolerance is associated with the disease called "gluten-sensitive enteropathy" or "**celiac disease**." It happens if your immune system responds abnormally to gluten, which is a part of wheat and some other grains. Some researchers include celiac disease as a food allergy. This abnormal immune system response, however, does not involve IgE antibody.

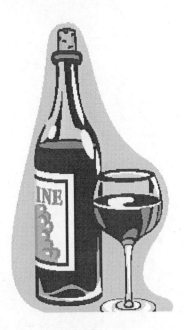

### Psychological causes

Some people may have a food intolerance that has a psychological trigger. If your food intolerance is caused by this type of trigger, a careful psychiatric evaluation may identify an unpleasant event in your life, often during childhood, tied to eating a particular food. Eating that food years later, even as an adult, is associated with a rush of unpleasant sensations.

### Other causes

There are several other conditions, including ulcers and cancers of the GI tract, that cause some of the same symptoms as food allergy. These symptoms include vomiting, diarrhea, and cramping abdominal pain made worse by eating.

## DIAGNOSIS

After ruling out food intolerances and other health problems, your healthcare provider will use several steps to find out if you have an allergy to specific foods.

## Detailed History

A detailed history is the most valuable tool for diagnosing food allergy. Your provider will ask you several questions and listen to your history of food reactions to decide if the facts fit a food allergy.

- What was the timing of your reaction?
- Did your reaction come on quickly, usually within an hour after eating the food?
- Did allergy medicines help? Antihistamines should relieve hives, for example.
- Is your reaction always associated with a certain food?
- Did anyone else who ate the same food get sick? For example, if you ate fish contaminated with histamine, everyone who ate the fish should be sick.
- How much did you eat before you had a reaction? The severity of a reaction is sometimes related to the amount of food eaten.
- How was the food prepared? Some people will have a violent allergic reaction only to raw or undercooked fish. Complete cooking of the fish may destroy the allergen, and they can then eat it with no allergic reaction.
- Did you eat other foods at the same time you had the reaction? Some foods may delay digestion and thus delay the start of the allergic reaction.

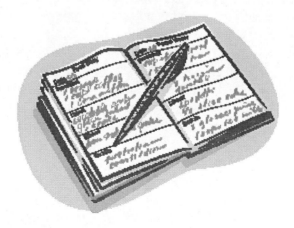

## Diet Diary

Sometimes your healthcare provider can't make a diagnosis solely on the basis of your history. In that case, you may be asked to record what you eat and whether you have a reaction. This diet diary gives more detail from which you and your provider can see if there is a consistent pattern in your reactions.

## Elimination Diet

The next step some healthcare providers use is an **elimination diet**. In this step, which is done under your provider's direction, certain foods are removed from your diet.

- You don't eat a food suspected of causing the allergy, such as eggs.
- You then substitute another food—in the case of eggs, another source of protein.

Your provider can almost always make a diagnosis if the symptoms go away after you remove the food from your diet. The diagnosis is confirmed if you then eat the food and the symptoms come back. You should do this only when the reactions are not significant and only under healthcare provider direction.

Your provider can't use this technique, however, if your reactions are severe or don't happen often. If you have a severe reaction, you should not eat the food again.

## Skin Test

If your history, diet diary, or elimination diet suggests a specific food allergy is likely, your healthcare provider will then use either the scratch or the prick skin test to confirm the diagnosis.

During a scratch skin test, your healthcare provider will place an **extract** of the food on the skin of your lower arm. Your provider will then scratch this portion of your skin with a needle and look for swelling or redness, which would be a sign of a local allergic reaction.

A prick skin test is done by putting a needle just below the surface of your skin of the lower arm. Then, a tiny amount of food extract is placed under the skin.

If the scratch or prick test is positive, it means that there is IgE on the skin's mast cells that is specific to the food being tested. Skin tests are rapid, simple, and relatively safe.

You can have a positive skin test to a food allergen, however, without having an allergic reaction to that food. A healthcare provider diagnoses a food allergy only when someone has a positive skin test to a specific allergen and when the history of reactions suggests an allergy to the same food.

## Blood Test

Your healthcare provider can make a diagnosis by doing a blood test as well. Indeed, if you are extremely allergic and have severe anaphylactic reactions, your provider can't use skin testing because causing an allergic reaction to the skin test could be dangerous. Skin testing also can't be done if you have eczema over a large portion of your body.

Your healthcare provider may use blood tests such as the RAST (radioallergosorbent test) and newer ones such as the CAP-RAST. Another blood test is called ELISA (enzymelinked immunosorbent **assay**). These blood tests measure the presence of food-specific IgE in your blood. The CAP-RAST can measure how much IgE your blood has to a specific food. As with skin testing, positive tests do not necessarily mean you have a food allergy.

## Double-Blind Oral Food Challenge

The final method healthcare providers use to diagnose food allergy is double-blind oral food **challenge**.

- Your healthcare provider will give you capsules containing individual doses of various foods, some of which are suspected of starting an allergic reaction. Or your provider will mask the suspected food within other foods known not to cause an allergic reaction.
- You swallow the capsules one at a time or swallow the masked food and are watched to see if a reaction occurs.

In a true double-blind test, your healthcare provider is also "blinded" (the capsules having been made up by another medical person). In that case your provider does not know which capsule contains the allergen.

The advantage of such a challenge is that if you react only to suspected foods and not to other foods tested, it confirms the diagnosis. You cannot be tested this way if you have a history of severe allergic reactions.

In addition, this testing is difficult because it takes a lot of time to perform and many food allergies are difficult to evaluate with this procedure. Consequently, many healthcare providers do not perform double-blind food challenges.

This type of testing is most commonly used if a healthcare provider thinks the reaction described is not due to a specific food and wishes to obtain evidence to support this. If your provider finds that your reaction is not due to a specific food, then additional efforts may be used to find the real cause of the reaction.

## TREATMENT

Food allergy is treated by avoiding the foods that trigger the reaction. Once you and your healthcare provider have identified the food(s) to which you are sensitive, you must remove them from your diet. To do this, you must read the detailed ingredient lists on each food you are considering eating.

Many allergy-producing foods such as peanuts, eggs, and milk, appear in foods one normally would not associate them with. Peanuts, for example, may be used as a protein source, and eggs are used in some salad dressings.

Because of a new law in the United States, FDA now requires ingredients in a packaged food to appear on its label. You can avoid most of the things to which you are sensitive if you read food labels carefully and avoid restaurant-prepared foods that might have ingredients to which you are allergic.

If you are highly allergic, even the tiniest amounts of a food allergen (for example, a small portion of a peanut kernel) can prompt an allergic reaction.

If you have food allergies, you must be prepared to treat unintentional exposure. Even people who know a lot about what they are sensitive to occasionally make a mistake. To protect yourself if you have had allergic reactions to a food, you should

- Wear a medical alert bracelet or necklace stating that you have a food allergy and are subject to severe reactions
- Carry an auto-injector device containing **epinephrine** (adrenaline), such as an epipen or twinject, that you can get by prescription and give to yourself if you think you are getting a food allergic reaction
- Seek medical help immediately, even if you have already given yourself epinephrine, by either calling the rescue squad or by getting transported to an emergency room

Anaphylactic allergic reactions can be fatal even when they start off with mild symptoms such as a tingling in the mouth and throat or GI discomfort.

---

### EXERCISE-INDUCED FOOD ALLERGY

At least one situation may require more than simply eating food with allergens to start a reaction: exercise-induced food allergy. People who have this reaction only experience it after eating a specific food before exercising. Some people get this reaction from many foods, and others get it only after eating a specific food. As exercise increases and body temperature rises, itching and light-headedness start and allergic reactions such as hives may appear and even anaphylaxis may develop.

The management of exercised-induced food allergy is simple—avoid eating for a couple of hours before exercising.

---

Schools and daycare centers must have plans in place to address any food allergy emergency. Parents and caregivers should take special care with children and learn how to

- Protect children from foods to which they are allergic
- Manage children if they eat a food to which they are allergic
- Give children epinephrine

Simply washing your hands with soap and water will remove peanut allergens. Also, most household cleaners will remove them from surfaces such as food preparation areas at home as well as daycare facilities and schools. These easy-to-do measures will help prevent peanut allergy reactions in children and adults.

There are several medicines you can take to relieve food allergy symptoms that are not part of an anaphylactic reaction. These include

- Antihistamines to relieve GI symptoms, hives, or sneezing and a runny nose
- Bronchodilators to relieve asthma symptoms

It is not easy to determine if a reaction to food is anaphylactic, however. It is important to develop a plan with a healthcare provider as to what reactions you should treat with epinephrine first, rather than antihistamines or bronchodilators.

## FOOD ALLERGY IN INFANTS AND CHILDREN

Allergy to cow's milk is particularly common in infants and young children. It causes hives and asthma in some children. In others, it can lead to colic and sleeplessness, and perhaps blood in the stool or poor growth. Infants are thought to be particularly susceptible to this allergic syndrome because their immune and digestive systems are immature. Milk allergy can develop within days to months of birth.

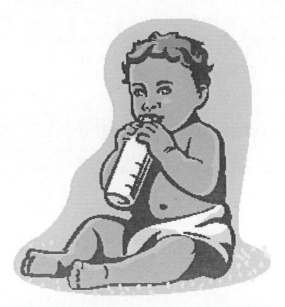

If your baby is on cow's milk formula, your healthcare provider may suggest a change to soy formula or an elemental formula if possible. Elemental formulas are produced from processed proteins with supplements added (basically sugars and **amino acids).** There are few if any allergens within these materials.

Healthcare providers sometimes prescribe **glucocorticosteroid** medicines to treat infants with very severe GI reactions to milk formulas. Fortunately, this food allergy tends to go away within the first few years of life.

Breast feeding often helps babies avoid feeding problems related to allergic reactions. Therefore, health experts often suggest that mothers feed their baby only breast milk for the first months of life to avoid milk allergy from developing within that timeframe.

Some babies are very sensitive to a certain food. If you are nursing and eat that food, sufficient amounts can enter your breast milk to cause a food reaction in your baby. To keep possible food allergens out of your breast milk, you might try not eating those foods, such as peanuts, that could cause an allergic reaction in your baby.

There is no conclusive evidence that breastfeeding prevents allergies from developing later in your child's life. It does, however, delay the start of food allergies by delaying your infant's exposure to those foods that can prompt allergies. Plus, it may avoid altogether food allergy problems sometimes seen in infants.

By delaying the introduction of solid foods until your baby is 6 months old or older, you can also prolong your baby's allergy-free period. Speak to your healthcare provider for specific instructions on when to add specific food groups to your child's diet.


# SOME CONTROVERSIAL AND UNPROVEN THEORIES

## Controversial and Unproven Disorders

There are several disorders that are popularly thought by some to be caused by food allergies. Either there is not enough scientific evidence to support those claims, or there is evidence that goes against such claims.

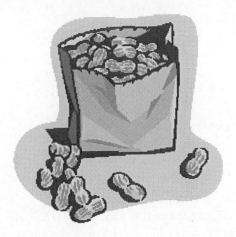

### Migraine headaches

There is controversy about whether migraine headaches can be caused by food allergy. Studies show people who are prone to migraines can have their headaches brought on by histamine and other substances in foods. The more difficult issue is whether food allergies actually cause migraines in such people.

### Arthritis

There is virtually no evidence that most rheumatoid arthritis or osteoarthritis can be made worse by foods, despite claims to the contrary.

### Allergic tension fatigue syndrome

There is no evidence that food allergies can cause a disorder called the allergic tension fatigue syndrome, in which people are tired, nervous, and may have problems concentrating or have headaches.

### Cerebral allergy

Cerebral allergy is a term that has been given to people who have trouble concentrating and have headaches as well as other complaints. These symptoms are sometimes blamed on mast cells activated in the brain but no other place in the body. Researchers have found no evidence that such a scenario can happen. Most health experts do not recognize cerebral allergy as a disorder.

*Environmental illness*

In a seemingly pristine environment, some people have many nonspecific complaints such as problems concentrating or depression. Sometimes this is blamed on small amounts of allergens or toxins in the environment. There is no evidence that these problems are due to food allergies.

*Childhood hyperactivity*

Some people believe hyperactivity in children is caused by food allergies. Researchers, however, have found that this behavioral disorder in children is only occasionally associated with food additives, and then only when such additives are consumed in large amounts.

There is no evidence that a true food allergy can affect a child's activity except for the possibility that if a child itches and sneezes and wheezes a lot, the child may be uncomfortable and therefore more difficult to guide. Also, children who are on anti-allergy medicines that cause drowsiness may get sleepy in school or at home.

## Controversial and Unproven Diagnostic Methods

*Cytotoxicity testing*

One controversial diagnostic technique is **cytotoxicity testing**, in which a food allergen is added to a blood sample. A technician then examines the sample under the microscope to see if white cells in the blood "die." Scientists have evaluated this technique in several studies and have found it does not effectively diagnose food allergy.

*Provocative challenge*

Another controversial approach is called sublingual (placed under the tongue) or subcutaneous (injected under the skin) **provocative challenge**. In this procedure, diluted food allergen is put under your tongue if you feel that your arthritis, for instance, is due to foods. The technician then asks you if the food allergen has made your arthritis symptoms worse. In clinical studies, researchers have not shown that this procedure can effectively diagnose food allergy.

> Sublingual provocative challenge is not the same as a potentially new treatment for food allergy called sublingual immunotherapy or SLIT. Researchers are currently evaluating this treatment.

### Immune complex assay

An immune complex assay is sometimes done on people suspected of having food allergies to see if groups, or complexes, of certain antibodies connect to the food allergen in the bloodstream. Some think that these immune groups link with food allergies. The formation of such immune complexes is a normal offshoot of food digestion, however, and everyone, if tested with a sensitive-enough measurement, has them. To date, no one has conclusively shown that this test links with allergies to foods.

### IgG subclass assay

Another test is the IgG subclass assay, which looks specifically for certain kinds of IgG antibody. Again, there is no evidence that this diagnoses food allergy.

## Controversial and Unproven Treatments

One controversial treatment, which sometimes may be used with provocative challenge, includes putting a diluted solution of a particular food under your tongue about a half hour before you eat the food suspected of causing an allergic reaction. This is an attempt to "neutralize" the subsequent exposure to the food you believe is harmful. The results of carefully conducted clinical research show this procedure does not prevent an allergic reaction.

### Allergy shots

Another unproven treatment involves getting allergy shots (immunotherapy) containing small quantities of the food extracts to which you are allergic. These shots are given regularly for a long period of time with the aim of "desensitizing" you to the food allergen. Researchers have not yet proven that allergy shots reliably relieve food allergies.

# RESEARCH

The National Institute of Allergy and Infectious Diseases conducts research on food allergy and other allergic diseases. This research is focused on understanding what happens to the body during the allergic process—the sequence of events leading to the allergic response and the factors responsible for allergic diseases. This understanding will lead to better methods of diagnosing, preventing, and treating allergic diseases. Researchers also are looking at better ways to study allergic reactions to foods.

Educating people, including patients, healthcare providers, school teachers, and daycare workers, about the importance of food allergy is also an important research focus. The more people know about the disorder, the better equipped they will be to control food allergies.

Several treatment approaches are currently being tested in research settings.

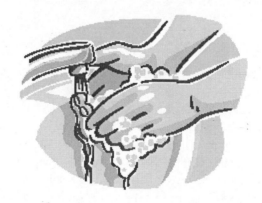

## Immunotherapy with Allergen Injections

One potential treatment for food allergy involves getting injections or shots (immunotherapy) subcutaneously (under the skin) that contain small quantities of the food extracts to which a person is allergic. These shots are given regularly for a long period of time with the aim of increasing the ability to tolerate the food allergen. Researchers have not yet found a safe and effective way to give allergens subcutaneously, because people often have allergic reactions to these injections.

## Immunotherapy with Allergen under the Tongue

Another potential treatment for food allergy involves putting allergens under the tongue, called sublingual immunotherapy (SLIT). Researchers think this is safer than giving under the skin. As of mid-2007, however, this treatment was only in very early stages.

## Anti-IgE Therapy

One published study suggested that some (but not all) people with peanut allergy might be partially protected against allergic reactions to low doses of peanut by taking regular subcutaneous injections of one particular form of a medicine called anti-IgE. Because the FDA-approved anti-IgE medicine has not yet been tested for peanut allergy, this treatment is not currently available for peanut allergy. Scientists need to do further research to determine the value of anti-IgE.

## MORE INFORMATION

**National Institute of Allergy and Infectious Diseases**
6610 Rockledge Drive, MSC 6612
Bethesda, MD 20892-6612
301–496–5717
www.niaid.nih.gov

**National Library of Medicine**
MedlinePlus
8600 Rockville Pike
Bethesda, MD 20894
1–888–FIND–NLM (1–888–346–3656) or 301–594–5983
www.medlineplus.gov

**American Academy of Allergy, Asthma & Immunology**
555 East Wells Street, Suite 1100
Milwaukee, WI 53202-3823

1–800–822–ASMA (1–800–822–2762)
www.aaaai.org

**The American Academy of Pediatrics**
141 Northwest Point Boulevard
Elk Grove Village, IL 60007-1098
847–434–4000
www.aap.org

**American College of Allergy, Asthma & Immunology**
85 West Algonquin Road, Suite 550
Arlington Heights, IL 60005
1–800–842–7777
www.acaai.org

**Asthma and Allergy Foundation of America**
1233 20th Street, NW, Suite 402
Washington, DC 20036
1–800–7–ASTHMA (1–800–727–8462) or 202–466–7643
www.aafa.org

**The Food Allergy and Anaphylaxis Network**
11781 Lee Jackson Highway, Suite 160
Fairfax, VA 22033
1–800–929–4040
www.foodallergy.org

## Allergy Extracts

**Food and Drug Administration**
**Center for Biologics Evaluation and Research**
1401 Rockville Pike
Rockville, MD 20852-1448
1–800–835–4709 or 301–827–1800
www,fda.gov/cber

## Celiac Disease and Lactose Intolerance

### National Institute of Diabetes and Digestive and Kidney Diseases
National Digestive Diseases Information Clearinghouse
2 Information Way
Bethesda, MD 20892-3570 1–800–891–5389
www.digestive.niddk.nih.gov

## Eczema

### National Arthritis and Musculoskeletal and Skin Diseases Information Clearinghouse
1 AMS Circle
Bethesda, MD 20892-3675
1–877–22–NIAMS (1–877–226–4267) or 301–495–4484
www.niams.nih.gov

### American Academy of Dermatology
P.O. Box 4014
Schaumburg, IL 60168-4014
847–330–0230
www.aad.org

### National Eczema Association for Science and Education
4460 Redwood Highway, Suite 16-D
San Rafael, CA 94903-1953
1–800–818–7546 or 415–499–3474
www.nationaleczema.org

## Food Contents

### U.S. Department of Agriculture
### Food and Nutrition Information Center
National Agricultural Library, Room 105
10301 Baltimore Avenue Beltsville, MD 20705-2351

301-504-5719
www.nal.usda.gov/finic


## Food Facts

**American Dietetic Association**
National Center for Nutrition and Dietetics Information Line
1–800–366–1655
www.eatright.org/Public


# GLOSSARY

**allergens**—substances that cause an allergic reaction.

**amino acids**—any of the 26 building blocks of proteins.

**anaphylaxis**—a severe reaction to an allergen that can cause itching, fainting, and in some cases, death.

**antibody**—a molecule tailor-made by the immune system to lock onto and destroy specific foreign substances such as allergens.

**assay**—a laboratory method of measuring a substance such as immunoglobulin.

**bacteria**—kind of microbe, some of which can contaminate or spoil food.

**basophils**—white blood cells that contribute to inflammatory reactions.

**challenge**—process of assessing the immune system's response to a food allergen.

**cells**—the smallest units of life; the basic living things that make up tissues.

**celiac disease**—a disease of the digestive system that damages the small intestine and interferes with absorption of nutritional contents of food.

**cytotoxicity testing**—an unproven laboratory method of diagnosing allergies by examining blood samples under a microscope to see if white blood cells "die."

**elimination diet**—certain foods are removed from a person's diet and a substitute food of the same type, such as another source of protein in place of eggs, is introduced.

**enzyme**—a protein produced by living cells that promotes specific biochemical reactions at body temperatures.

**epinephrine**—a drug form of adrenaline (a natural hormone in the body) that stimulates nerves.

**extract**—a concentrated liquid preparation containing minute parts of specific foods.

**gastrointestinal (GI) tract**—an area of the body that includes the stomach and intestines.

**glucocorticoid**—a type of steroid drug that reduces inflammation.

**granule**—grain-like part of a cell.

**histamine**—chemical released by mast cells and basophils.

**histamine toxicity**—an allergic-like reaction to eating foods containing high levels of histamine.

**immune system**—a complex network of specialized cells, tissues, and organs, such as the lungs, that defends the body against attacks by disease-causing microbes.

**immunoglobulin**—one of a large family of proteins, also known as antibody.

**inflammation**—an immune system reaction to allergens or germs. Signs include redness, swelling, pain, or heat.

**lactose intolerance**—the inability to digest lactose, a kind of sugar found in milk and other food products. Lactose intolerance is caused by a shortage of the enzyme lactase, which is produced by the cells that line the small intestine.

**microbes**—tiny life forms, such as bacteria, viruses, and fungi, that may cause disease.

**mast cells**—large granule-containing cells found in body tissues that are typical sites of allergic reactions.

**molecule**—building block of a cell; examples are proteins, fats, and carbohydrates.

**provocative challenge**—an unproven test in which diluted food allergen is placed under the tongue or injected under the skin to find out whether symptoms get worse.

**tissues**—groups of similar cells joined to perform the same function.

**toxins**—agents produced by plants and bacteria that are poisonous and that also may trigger allergic reactions.

In: Food Allergy Overview and Children's...          ISBN: 978-1-61728-478-6
Editor: Lee R. Daniels                    © 2010 Nova Science Publishers, Inc.

*Chapter 2*

# FOOD ALLERGIES: REDUCING THE RISKS*

## *FDA Consumer Health Information*

Food allergies can range from merely irritating to life-threatening. Approximately 30,000 Americans go to the emergency room each year to get treated for severe food allergies, according to the Food Allergy and Anaphylaxis Network (FAAN). It is estimated that 150 to 200 Americans die each year because of allergic reactions to food.

Food allergies affect about two percent of adults and four to eight percent of children in the United States, and the number of young people with food allergies has increased over the last decade, according to a recent report by the Centers for Disease Control and Prevention (CDC). Children with food allergies are more likely to have asthma, eczema, and other types of allergies.

Some food allergies can be outgrown. Studies have shown that the severity of food allergies can change throughout a person's life.

"There is no cure for food allergies," says Stefano Luccioli, M.D., senior medical advisor in the Food and Drug Administration's (FDA) Office of Food Additive Safety (OFAS). "The best way for consumers to protect themselves is by avoiding food items that will cause a reaction." OFAS is part of FDA's Center for Food Safety and Applied Nutrition (CFSAN).

---

* This is an edited, reformatted and augmented version of a Food and Drug Administration publication dated January 2009.

To reduce the risks from allergic reactions, FDA is working to ensure that major allergenic ingredients in food are accurately labeled in accordance with the Food Allergen Labeling and Consumer Protection Act of 2004 (FALCPA). Allergenic ingredients are substances that are capable of causing an allergic reaction.

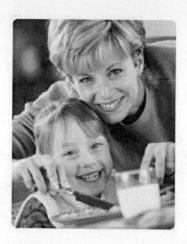

In addition, there has been widespread use of allergen advisory labels on products that may have allergenic ingredients that were introduced by way of cross contact during the manufacturing process. Cross contact occurs when a residue or other trace amount of an allergenic food is unintentionally incorporated into another food.

Because FALPCA does not require the declaration of allergenic ingredients introduced through cross contact, FDA is developing a long-term strategy that will help manufacturers use voluntary allergen advisory labeling that:

- Is not misleading
- Conveys a clear and uniform message
- Adequately informs food-allergic consumers and their caregivers

## WHAT IS A FOOD ALLERGY?

A food allergy is a specific type of adverse food reaction involving the immune system. The body produces what is called an allergic, or immunoglobulin E (IgE), antibody to a food. Once a specific food is ingested and binds with the IgE antibody, an allergic response ensues.

A food allergy should not be confused with a food intolerance or other nonallergic food reactions. Various epidemiological surveys have indicated that almost 80 percent of people who are asked if they have a food allergy respond that they do when, in fact, they do not have a true IgE-mediated food allergy.

Food intolerance refers to an abnormal response to a food or additive, but it differs from an allergy in that it does not involve the immune system. For example, people who have recurring gastrointestinal problems when they drink milk may say they have a milk allergy. But they really may be lactose intolerant.

"One of the main differences between food allergies and food intolerances is that food allergies can result in an immediate, life-threatening response," says Luccioli. "Thus, compared to food intolerances, food allergic reactions pose a much greater health risk."

## SIGNS AND SYMPTOMS

Symptoms of a food allergy usually develop within about an hour after eating the offending food. The most common signs and symptoms of a food allergy include:

- Hives, itching, or skin rash
- Swelling of the lips, face, tongue and throat, or other parts of the body
- Wheezing, nasal congestion, or trouble breathing
- Abdominal pain, diarrhea, nausea, or vomiting
- Dizziness, lightheadedness, or fainting

In a severe allergic reaction to food—called anaphylaxis—you may have more extreme versions of the above reactions. Or you may experience life-threatening signs and symptoms such as:

- Swelling of the throat and air passages that makes it difficult to breathe
- Shock, with a severe drop in blood pressure
- Rapid, irregular pulse
- Loss of consciousness

# Major Food Allergens

FALCPA, a comprehensive food labeling law, has been in effect since January 1, 2006.

Under FALCPA, food labels are required to state clearly whether the food contains a major food allergen.

A major food allergen is defined as one of the following foods or food groups, or is an ingredient that contains protein derived from one of the following foods or food groups:

- Milk
- Eggs
- Peanuts
- Tree nuts such as almonds, walnuts, and pecans
- Soybeans
- Wheat
- Fish
- Shellfish such as crab, lobster, and shrimp

"These foods or food groups account for 90 percent of all food allergies in the United States, and FALCPA focuses on IgE-related food allergies," according to Luccioli. "This law does not protect everyone with a food allergy, but should protect the majority of people who may have severe allergic responses to foods," he says.

More than 160 different foods have been reported to cause allergies; the list of major allergens in the United States is limited to eight foods. "Other countries may have different foods on their lists because food allergies reflect patterns of consumption," Luccioli says. "For example, in Europe there is a high prevalence of allergies to mustard and celery."

# FDA Public Hearing on Labeling

FDA held a public hearing on September 16, 2008, to help the agency determine how manufacturers use advisory labeling for food allergens.

FDA is also evaluating how consumers interpret different advisory labeling statements, as well as what wording is likely to be most effective in communicating the likelihood that an allergen may be present in a food.

"The public hearing was held in part to address labeling that manufacturers voluntarily use because of cross contact concerns," says Felicia Billingslea, director of the Food Labeling and Standards Staff in FDA's Office of Nutrition, Labeling and Dietary Supplements.

Cross contact may occur during:

- Harvesting
- Transportation
- Manufacturing
- Processing
- Storage

Many food manufacturers may try to prevent cross contact through the use of dedicated facilities or dedicated production lines. Also, a variety of advisory statements are used on package labels to indicate possible cross contact. For example, a label might indicate: "Produced in a plant that processes wheat."

FDA asked twelve questions at the public hearing that related to the use of specific advisory statements and advisory labeling in general.

Some of the questions asked were:

- What specific advisory statements adequately inform consumers of the potential risk of cross contact with allergenic materials?
- What advisory statements most accurately communicate to consumers and their caregivers the potential risk of the presence of an allergen? Why?

## ADVICE FOR CONSUMERS

If you have food allergies, you must be prepared for unintentional exposures. To protect yourself, the National Institute of Allergies and Infectious Diseases (NIAID) recommends that you:

- Wear a medical alert bracelet or necklace stating that you have a food allergy and are subject to severe reactions.
- Carry an auto-injector device containing epinephrine (adrenaline) that you can get by prescription and give to yourself if you think you are experiencing a food allergic reaction.

- Seek medical help immediately if you experience a food allergic reaction, even if you have already given yourself epinephrine, either by calling 911 or getting transportation to an emergency room.

This article appears on FDA's Consumer Health Information Web page (www.fda.gov/consumer), which features the latest updates on FDA-regulated products. Sign up for free e-mail subscriptions at www.fda.gov/consumer/consumerenews.html.

## For More Information

CFSAN Food Labeling and Nutrition page
www.foodsafety.gov/label.html

CFSAN Information About Food Allergies
www.cfsan.fda.gov/~dms/wh-alrgy.html

The Food Allergy and Anaphylaxis Network
www.foodallergy.org/

CDC Press Release: Study on Food Allergies in Children
www.cdc.gov/media/pressrel/2008/r081022.htm

In: Food Allergy Overview and Children's... ISBN: 978-1-61728-478-6
Editor: Lee R. Daniels © 2010 Nova Science Publishers, Inc.

*Chapter 3*

# FOOD ALLERGY AMONG U.S. CHILDREN: TRENDS IN PREVALENCE AND HOSPITALIZATIONS*

## *Amy M. Branum and Susan L. Lukacs*
U.S. Department of Health and Human Services,
Centers for Disease Control and Prevention

## KEY FINDINGS

- In 2007, approximately 3 million children under age 18 years (3.9%) were reported to have a food or digestive allergy in the previous 12 months.
- From 1997 to 2007, the prevalence of reported food allergy increased 18% among children under age 18 years.
- Children with food allergy are two to four times more likely to have other related conditions such as asthma and other allergies, compared with children without food allergies.
- From 2004 to 2006, there were approximately 9,500 hospital discharges per year with a diagnosis related to food allergy among children under age 18 years.

---

* This is an edited, reformatted and augmented version of a National Center for Health Statistics publication dated October 2008.

**Note: See Definitions for an explanation of reported food allergy.**

Food allergy is a potentially serious immune response to eating specific foods or food additives. Eight types of food account for over 90% of allergic reactions in affected individuals: milk, eggs, peanuts, tree nuts, fish, shellfish, soy, and wheat [1,2]. Reactions to these foods by an allergic person can range from a tingling sensation around the mouth and lips and hives to death, depending on the severity of the allergy. The mechanisms by which a person develops an allergy to specific foods are largely unknown. Food allergy is more prevalent in children than adults, and a majority of affected children will "outgrow" food allergies with age. However, food allergy can sometimes become a lifelong concern [1]. Food allergies can greatly affect children and their families' well-being. There are some indications that the prevalence of food allergy may be increasing in the United States and in other countries [2–4].

**Keywords:** *allergy • National Health Interview Survey • National Hospital Discharge Survey*

## FOUR OUT OF EVERY 100 CHILDREN HAVE A FOOD ALLERGY

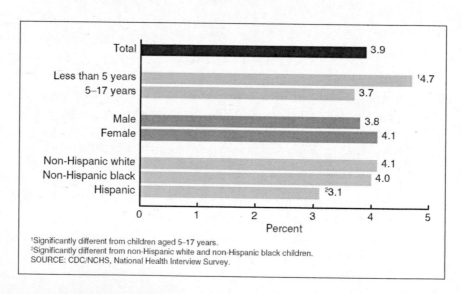

Figure 1. Percentage of children under age 18 years who had a reported food or digestive allergy in the past 12 months, by age, sex, and race and ethnicity group:

In 2007, an estimated 3 million children under age 18 years (3.9%) had a reported food allergy.

Children under age 5 years had higher rates of reported food allergy compared with children 5 to 17 years of age. Boys and girls had similar rates of food allergy.

Hispanic children had lower rates of reported food allergy than non-Hispanic white or non-Hispanic black children.

## FOOD ALLERGY AMONG CHILDREN IN THE UNITED STATES IS BECOMING MORE COMMON OVER TIME

In 2007, the reported food allergy rate among all children younger than 18 years was 18% higher than in 1997. During the 10-year period 1997 to 2006, food allergy rates increased significantly among both preschool-aged and older children.

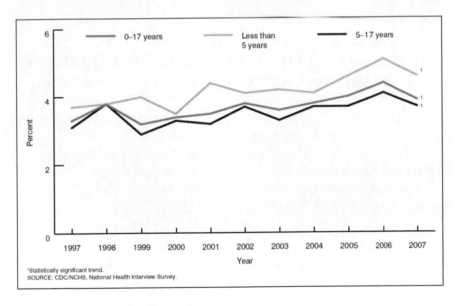

Figure 2. Percentage of children under age 18 years who had a reported food or digestive allergy in the past 12 months, by age group: United States, 1997–2007

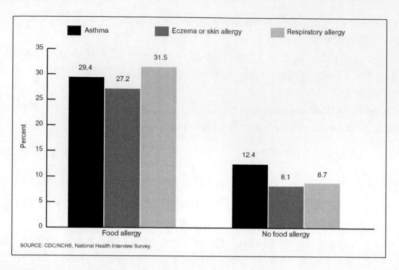

Figure 3. Percentage of children under age 18 years with asthma or other reported allergic conditions in the previous 12 months, by reported food allergy status: United States, 2007

## CHILDREN WITH FOOD ALLERGY ARE MORE LIKELY TO HAVE ASTHMA OR OTHER ALLERGIC CONDITIONS

In 2007, 29% of children with food allergy also had reported asthma compared with 12% of children without food allergy.

Approximately 27% of children with food allergy had reported eczema or skin allergy, compared with 8% of children without food allergy.

Over 30% of children with food allergy also had reported respiratory allergy, compared with 9% of children with no food

## RECENT DATA SHOW HOSPITALIZATIONS WITH DIAGNOSES RELATED TO FOOD ALLERGIES HAVE INCREASED AMONG CHILDREN

From 2004 to 2006, there were an average of 9,537 hospital discharges per year with a diagnosis related to food allergy among children 0 to 17 years.

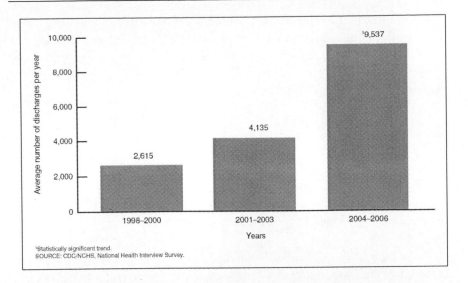

Figure 4. Average number of hospital discharges per year among children under age 18 years with any diagnosis related to food allergy: United States, 1998–2006

Hospital discharges with a diagnosis related to food allergy increased significantly over time from 1998–2000 through 2004–2006.

## SUMMARY

Reported food allergy has increased among children of all ages in the United States over the last 10 years. Nationally representative survey data corroborates reports of increasing food allergy in the United States, and our findings are similar to those reported in other countries. There is some difference in reported food allergy according to Hispanic ethnicity, with lower reported rates among Hispanic children compared with non-Hispanic white and non-Hispanic black children. However, reported food allergy does not appear to differ by sex.

Children with food allergy are two to four times as likely to experience other allergic conditions and asthma than children without food allergy. This is of great importance as children with coexisting food allergy and asthma may be more likely to experience anaphylactic reactions to foods and be at higher risk of death [5,6].

Hospitalizations having at least one diagnosis related to food allergy also increased from 1998–2000 through 2004–2006. This finding could be related to increased awareness, reporting, and use of specific medical diagnostic codes for food allergy or could represent a real increase in children who are experiencing food-allergic reactions.

# DEFINITIONS

*Reported food allergy, National Health Interview Survey (NHIS):* is defined by an affirmative answer to the question "During the past 12 months, has (child) had any kind of food or digestive allergy?"

*Food allergy diagnosis, National Hospital Discharge Survey (NHDS)*: is defined by the *International Classification of Diseases, Ninth Revision, Clinical Modification* (ICD–9–CM) codes relevant to food allergy and anaphylaxis related to food allergy.

*Reported asthma (NHIS):* is defined by an affirmative answer to the question "Has a doctor or health professional ever told you that (child) had asthma?"

*Reported eczema or skin allergy (NHIS):* is defined by an affirmative answer to the question "During the past 12 months, has (child) had eczema or any kind of skin allergy?"

*Reported respiratory allergy (NHIS):* is defined by an affirmative answer to the question "During the past 12 months, has (child) had any kind of respiratory allergy?"

# DATA SOURCE AND METHODS

The National Health Interview Survey (NHIS) was used in this analysis to estimate the prevalence of food allergy among children in the United States. The NHIS is a multipurpose health survey conducted by the Centers for Disease Control and Prevention's National Center for Health Statistics, and is the principal source of information on the health of the civilian, noninstitutionalized, household population of the United States. The NHIS consists of a Basic Module and variable Supplements. The Basic Module, which remains largely unchanged from year to year, consists of three components: the Family Core, the Sample Child Core, and the Sample Adult Core. Questions from the child core related to food allergy, asthma, and other allergic conditions were used for this analysis. The 2007 NHIS questionnaire containing these questions can be viewed at: http://www.cdc.gov/ nchs/nhis.htm.

The NHIS uses a multistage sample designed to represent the civilian noninstitutionalized population of the United States. In 2007, approximately 9,500 children were sampled. Each sampled child is assigned a weight in order to reflect their representation of the U.S. child population. In order to make estimates on a national level, it is necessary to utilize the person's basic assigned sampling weight for proper analysis. Therefore, the data for this analysis were weighted to make national estimates.

The National Hospital Discharge Survey (NHDS) was used in this analysis to estimate the number of hospital discharges among children attributable to food allergy. The NHDS is a national probability survey designed to meet the need for information on characteristics of inpatients discharged from nonfederal short-stay hospitals in the United States. The NHDS collects data from a sample of approximately 270,000 inpatient records acquired from a national sample of about 500 hospitals. Only hospitals with an average length of stay of fewer than 30 days for all patients, general hospitals, or children's general hospitals are included in the survey. Federal, military, and Department of Veterans Affairs hospitals, as well as hospital units of institutions (such as prison hospitals), and hospitals with fewer than six beds staffed for patient use, are excluded.

The NHDS uses a three-stage sampling design procedure to produce national estimates of hospital discharges. Weights are assigned to each sample record. When used collectively, the sample is representative of the United States. A maximum of seven diagnostic codes was assigned for each sample abstract. Further information about the NHDS can be found at: http://www.cdc.gov/nchs/about/major/hdasd/nhds.htm.

The ICD–9–CM codes used to identify food allergy in the NHDS included 477.1 (allergic rhinitis due to food), 558.3 (allergic gastroenteritis and colitis), 692.5 (contact dermatitis due to food in contact with skin), 693.1 (dermatitis due to food taken internally), 995.6 (anaphylactic shock due to adverse food reaction with specific codes for unspecified food, peanuts, crustaceans, fruits and vegetables, tree nuts and seeds, fish, food additives, milk products, eggs, other specified food), and 995.7 (other adverse food reactions not elsewhere classified). Trend tests were performed to evaluate changes in reported food allergy over time using weighted least squares regression. Chi-square tests were performed to evaluate differences in food allergy between groups. All estimates shown have an unweighted sample size of 30 or greater and a relative standard error less than or equal to 30%. All significance tests were two-sided using $p < 0.05$ as the level of statistical significance. Terms such as "similar" indicate that the statistics being compared were not statistically significant. All data analyses were performed using the statistical packages SAS version 9.1 (SAS Institute, Cary, N.C.) and STATA.

## ABOUT THE AUTHORS

Amy M. Branum and Susan L. Lukacs are with the Centers for Disease Control and Prevention's National Center for Health Statistics, Office of Analysis and Epidemiology, Infant, Child, and Women's Health Statistics Branch.

## REFERENCES

[1]   Sampson, H A. (2004). Update on food allergy. *J Allergy Clin Immunol, 113*, 805–19.
[2]   Sicherer, S.H. (2002). Food allergy. *Lancet, 360,* 701–10.
[3]   Sicherer, S.H., Munoz-Furlong, A. & Sampson, H.A. (2003). Prevalence of peanut and tree nut allergy in the United States determined by means of random digit dial telephone survey: a 5–year follow-up study. *J Allergy Clin Immunol, 112,* 1203–7.
[4]   Grundy, J. Matthews, S. Bateman, B. Dean, T. & Arshad, S.H. (2002). Rising prevalence of allergy to peanut in children: data from 2 sequential cohorts. *J Allergy Clin Immunol, 110,*784–9.
[5]   Bock, S.A, Munoz-Furlong, A. & Sampson, H.A. (2007). Further fatalities caused by anaphylactic reactions to food, 2001–2006. *J Allergy Clin Immunol, 119,*1016–18.
[6]   Colver, A.F., Nevantaus, H., Macdougall, C.F. & Cant, A.J. (2005). Severe food-allergic reactions in children across the UK and Ireland, 1998–2000. *Acta Paediatr, 94,* 689–95.

**Suggested citation**
Branum AM, Lukacs SL. Food allergy among U.S. children: Trends in prevalence and hospitalizations. NCHS data brief, no 10. Hyattsville, MD: National Center for Health Statistics. 2008.

**National Center for Health Statistics**
Director
Edward J. Sondik, Ph.D.
Acting Co-Deputy Directors
Jennifer H. Madans, Ph.D. Michael H. Sadagursky

In: Food Allergy Overview and Children's...       ISBN: 978-1-61728-478-6
Editor: Lee R. Daniels                    © 2010 Nova Science Publishers, Inc.

*Chapter 4*

# FOOD ALLERGIES: WHAT YOU NEED TO KNOW[*]

## U.S. Food and Drug Administration

*Each year, millions of Americans have allergic reactions to food. Although most food allergies cause relatively mild and minor symptoms, some food allergies can cause severe reactions, and may even be life-threatening.*

*There is no cure for food allergies. Strict avoidance of food allergens — and early recognition and management of allergic reactions to food — are important measures to prevent serious health consequences.*

## FDA'S ROLE

### New Labeling for 2006

To help Americans avoid the health risks posed by food allergens, Congress passed the **Food Allergen Labeling and Consumer Protection Act of 2004**. The new law applies to all foods regulated by FDA, both domestic and imported, that are labeled on or after January 1, 2006. (FDA regulates all foods except meat, poultry, and certain egg products.)

---

[*] This is an edited, reformatted and augmented version of a Food and Drug Administration publication dated February 2007.

- Before the new law, the labels of foods made from two or more ingredients were required to list all **ingredients** by their common, or usual, names. The names of some ingredients, however, do not clearly identify their source.
- Now, the labels required by the new law must clearly identify the **source** of all ingredients that are — or are derived from — the **eight most common food allergens**.

As a result, food labels will help allergic consumers to identify offending foods or ingredients so they can more easily avoid them.

## ABOUT FOODS LABELED *BEFORE* JANUARY 1, 2006

Food products labeled *before* January 1, 2006 were not required to be re-labeled under the new law. However, these foods may still be on store shelves — so be sure to take that into consideration while shopping, and always use special care when reading labels.

## FOOD ALLERGIES: WHAT TO DO *IF SYMPTOMS OCCUR*

The appearance of symptoms (see *Know the Symptoms* at right) after eating food may be a sign of a food allergy. The food(s) that caused these symptoms should be avoided, and the affected person, should contact a doctor or health care provider for appropriate testing and evaluation.

- Persons found to have a food allergy should be taught to **read labels** and **avoid the offending foods**. They should also be taught, in case of accidental ingestion, to **recognize the early symptoms** of an allergic reaction, and be properly educated on — and armed with — appropriate treatment measures.
- Persons with a known food allergy who begin experiencing symptoms while, or after, eating a food should **initiate treatment immediately**, and go to a **nearby emergency room** if symptoms progress.

# WHAT ARE MAJOR FOOD ALLERGENS?

While more than 160 foods can cause allergic reactions in people with food allergies, the new law identifies the eight most common allergenic foods. These foods account for 90 percent of food allergic reactions, and are the food sources from which many other ingredients are derived.

*The* **eight foods identified by the law are:**

1. **Milk**
2. **Eggs**
3. **Fish** (e.g., bass, flounder, cod)
4. **Crustacean shellfish** (e.g., crab, lobster, shrimp)
5. **Tree nuts** (e.g., almonds, walnuts, pecans)
6. **Peanuts**
7. **Wheat**
8. **Soybeans**

These eight foods, and any ingredient that contains protein derived from one or more of them, are designated as "major food allergens" by the new law.

## How Major Food *Allergens* Are Listed

The new law requires that food labels identify the food source of all major food allergens. Unless the food source of a major food allergen is part of the ingredient's common or usual name (or is already identified in the ingredient list), it must be included in **one of two ways**.

The name of the food source of a major food allergen must appear:

1. **In parentheses** following the name of the ingredient.
   *Examples:* "lecithin (soy)," "flour (wheat)," and "whey (milk)"

— OR —

2. **Immediately after or next to** the list of ingredients in a "contains" statement.
   *Example*: "Contains Wheat, Milk, and Soy."

# KNOW THE SYMPTOMS

Symptoms of food allergies typically appear from within a few minutes to two hours after a person has eaten the food to which he or she is allergic.

**Allergic reactions can include:**
- Hives
- Flushed skin or rash
- Tingling or itchy sensation in the mouth
- Face, tongue, or lip swelling
- Vomiting and/or diarrhea
- Abdominal cramps
- Coughing or wheezing
- Dizziness and/or lightheadedness
- Swelling of the throat and vocal cords
- Difficulty breathing
- Loss of consciousness

## About Other Allergens

Persons may still be allergic to — and have serious reactions to — foods other than the eight foods identified by the new law. So, always be sure to read the food label's ingredient list carefully to avoid the food allergens in question.

# THE HARD FACTS

## Severe Food Allergies Can Be Life-Threatening

Following ingestion of a food allergen(s), a person with food allergies can experience a severe, life-threatening allergic reaction called **anaphylaxis**.

*This can lead to:*
- constricted airways in the lungs
- severe lowering of blood pressure and shock ("**anaphylactic shock**")
- suffocation by swelling of the throat

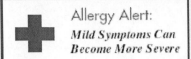

Allergy Alert:
*Mild Symptoms Can Become More Severe*

Initially mild *symptoms* that occur after ingesting a food allergen are not always a measure of mild *severity*. In fact, if not treated promptly, these symptoms can become more serious in a very short amount of time, and could lead to anaphylaxis. See *The Hard Facts* at left.

Each year in the U.S., it is estimated that anaphylaxis to food results in:

- 30,000 emergency room visits
- 2,000 hospitalizations
- 150 deaths

Prompt administration of epinephrine by autoinjector (e.g., Epi-pen) during early symptoms of anaphylaxis may help prevent these serious consequences.

In: Food Allergy Overview and Children's...        ISBN: 978-1-61728-478-6
Editor: Lee R. Daniels                © 2010 Nova Science Publishers, Inc.

*Chapter 5*

# REPORT OF THE NIH EXPERT PANEL ON FOOD ALLERGY RESEARCH*

## *National Institute of Allergy and Infectious Diseases*

### OBJECTIVE

The Food Allergen and Consumer Protection Act of 2004 (Public Law 108-282) requires the Secretary of Health and Human Services, acting through the Director of the National Institutes of Health (NIH), to convene an *ad hoc* panel of experts in allergy and immunology to review current basic and clinical research efforts related to food allergies, and requires that the panel make recommendations to the Secretary for enhancing and coordinating research activities concerning food allergies.

At the request of the NIH Director, the National Institute of Allergy and Infectious Diseases (NIAID) convened the NIH Expert Panel on Food Allergy Research in March 2006 as a working group of the National Advisory Allergy and Infectious Disease Council. Dr. Dean D. Metcalfe (NIAID, NIH) and Dr. Stephen J. Galli (Stanford University) co-chaired a nineteen-member panel of national and international experts. Other participants included representatives of various federal agencies, professional societies, advocacy groups and

---

* This is an edited, reformatted and augmented version of a National Institutes of Health publication dated March 2006.

organizations, as well as interested individuals. The roster of the expert panel members and a list of panel observers are in **Appendix A**; the meeting agenda is in **Appendix B**.

The Expert Panel meeting began with a series of overview presentations, including an NIAID staff presentation reviewing the current NIAID research portfolio, followed by ten breakout sessions focused on key topics relevant to food allergy research. The presentations and breakout sessions referenced key scientific publications that are relevant to advances in food allergy research and development of research recommendations. The Panel held summary sessions to integrate and prioritize the recommendations of each breakout session.

This report summarizes the findings and recommendations of the Expert Panel.

# BACKGROUND

Food allergy is an immunologic disease responsible for significant morbidity. In the United States, the prevalence of food allergy is 6–8 percent of children under four years of age, and is 3.7 percent of adults. The prevalence of food allergy appears to be increasing, with allergies to peanut increasing substantially. Food allergy is frequently accompanied by other allergic diseases including atopic dermatitis (eczema) and asthma, and asthma is an important risk factor for severe allergic reactions to food. Patients with food allergy may have mild reactions, such as hives, but are also at risk for anaphylaxis, a severe and life-threatening systemic allergic reaction characterized by hives, fall of blood pressure, upper airway obstruction, and severe wheezing. Food allergy accounts for about 35–50 percent of emergency room visits for anaphylaxis and causes about 30,000 episodes of anaphylaxis and 100–200 deaths per year in the United States. Even with assiduous avoidance of known food allergens, each year approximately one of every four food allergic individuals will have an accidental exposure that leads to a food-induced reaction. Severe, life-threatening reactions occur mostly in adolescents and young adults, and peanuts and tree nuts are the most common causes of such reactions. Currently, the only treatments for food allergy are allergen avoidance and management of reactions caused by allergen exposure. In addition to the psychological effects of the risk of death and the stigma of avoiding common foods, food allergy has nutritional impacts on the health, development, and lifestyle of children.

Hence, food allergy has emerged as an important public health problem based on its increasing prevalence, persistence throughout life for those who are sensitized to the foods most likely to cause severe reactions (peanut and tree nut), the potential for fatal reactions, and lack of preventive treatment other than food avoidance.

Physicians base the diagnosis of food allergy primarily on the clinical history. Confirmatory information can be obtained by blood tests or skin prick tests that detect allergic (IgE) antibodies to food allergens. The most definitive diagnostic test is a double-blind, placebo-controlled food challenge (DBPCFC) in which patients are fed increasing amounts of the foods in question in a carefully monitored clinical research environment. When conducted by experienced clinical investigators, the risks can be minimized, but a DBPCFC is still associated with the potential for severe allergic reactions, raising complex questions about its use in clinical research. Those issues are addressed elsewhere in this document.

## Overview of Food Allergic Reactions

Food allergy is defined as an immune-mediated adverse reaction to food. In allergic individuals, certain foods trigger the immune system to produce a characteristic class of antibodies against the allergen, called immunoglobulin E (IgE). IgE binds to receptors that are present on the surfaces of two types of cells—mast cells, which are present in the tissues; and basophils, which circulate in the blood. When an individual who has been sensitized to a particular allergen is re-exposed to that allergen, the allergen binds to IgE on these cells, triggering them to release potent mediators of allergic inflammation including histamine, leukotrienes, and protein messengers known as cytokines. These mediators stimulate the accumulation of eosinophils, a type of white blood cell that is characteristic of allergic inflammation. The mediators are also responsible for the appearance of allergic symptoms. For example, histamine triggers leakage of fluid from small blood vessels into the tissues, and it causes smooth muscle to contract. In mild allergic reactions, leakage of small amounts of fluid into the skin contributes to hives, or urticaria. In severe allergic reactions, leakage of larger volumes of fluid from the circulatory system can cause the blood pressure to drop. Contraction of smooth muscles in the larynx and trachea cuts off airflow. Contraction of smooth muscles in the lung contributes to bronchoconstriction and wheezing, signs of severe asthma. Antihistamines block the effects of low and moderate concentrations of histamine and can be effective in treating mild allergic reactions, especially hives. Because severe allergic reactions generate high concentrations of histamine and other mediators that are not blocked by antihistamines, antihistamines are far less effective in severe reactions. The most effective therapy for severe allergic reactions is epinephrine, which reverses the effects of histamine and other mediators on blood vessels and smooth muscle, and also blocks the continued release of mediators from mast cells and basophils.

Production of IgE antibodies is a complex process involving sequential cellular interactions involving several types of cells of the immune system including antigen-presenting cells, which engulf the allergens and present them to the immune system, and T and B lymphocytes. In allergic individuals, a subset of T lymphocytes produces certain cytokines that induce B lymphocytes to produce IgE in addition to other classes of antibodies. Other cytokines are potent inhibitors of IgE synthesis. The balance of these T cell-derived cytokines in a given individual contributes to the likelihood of becoming sensitized and having allergic symptoms.

# CURRENT STATUS AND RECENT ADVANCES IN FOOD ALLERGY RESEARCH

## Overview of NIH-Sponsored Food Allergy Research

NIH is the major source of federal funding for basic, translational, and clinical research on food allergy. Within NIH, NIAID is the designated lead institute, although other NIH Institutes (e.g., the National Institute of Diabetes and Digestive and Kidney Diseases) support basic research relevant to food allergy research, such as immunology of the gastrointestinal tract. NIAID convened expert panels to review food allergy research in 1996 and 2003, and the current panel in 2006.

The NIAID food allergy research portfolio has expanded substantially since the last expert panel review. This portfolio includes several single investigator-directed projects; a multi-investigator program project grant on milk allergy; and a consortium of food allergy researchers (CoFAR) that conducts pre-clinical research and clinical trials. In addition to these projects, the NIAID-sponsored Inner-City Asthma Consortium (ICAC) is conducting an observational study of children, enrolled at birth, who are at high risk for development of allergic diseases. NIAID also supports a wide range of basic research projects on fundamental immunology, allergic mechanisms, and mucosal immunology that will undoubtedly facilitate progress in food allergy research.

In FY 2006, NIAID will open two clinical trials to prevent food allergy and other allergic diseases through another clinical research program, the Immune Tolerance Network (ITN). The clinical trials conducted by CoFAR, ICAC, and the ITN are outlined later in this report in the section on clinical research. Recent and future year planned initiatives focusing on food allergy research are briefly outlined in the following paragraphs.

- In FY 2005, NIAID initiated CoFAR with planned support for five years, plus additional support dedicated to a CoFAR statistical and clinical coordinating center. This initiative addresses recommendations of the 2003 NIH Expert Panel on Food Allergy Research and will support: 1) preclinical research; 2) observational studies and immune-based interventions for treatment or prevention; and 3) the development, implementation, and dissemination of educational programs for children, their parents, and pediatric healthcare workers.
- In FY 2007, NIAID will initiate a program called "The Allergen and T Cell Reagent Resources for the Study of Allergic Diseases," which will provide new understanding of allergen structure and make novel reagents available to the research community. NIAID anticipates that some of the funded studies will be directly relevant to food allergens.
- In 2004 and 2005, NIAID and the Food Allergy and Anaphylaxis Network cosponsored a series of conferences on the definition and management of anaphylaxis. The conference reports were published in leading journals and provided opinions of international experts on the definition and management of anaphylaxis and an outline of a proposed research agenda.

The Panel discussed a number of challenges that NIH faces in expanding support for food allergy research. Chief among them is the small cadre of academic investigators working in this arena. Any sustained expansion of the research effort will require bringing new investigators into the field, a challenging prospect in an era of tight fiscal constraints. Furthermore, the recent growth in food allergy research has been highly leveraged through solicited research programs, as opposed to intrinsic growth in the number of investigator-initiated research project grants. In this regard, only 15 percent of the current NIAID support for food allergy research is through investigator-initiated awards, compared to approximately 60 percent of investigator-initiated awards for the full spectrum of NIAID-supported research on immunology and immune-mediated diseases. The solicited research programs in food allergy include CoFAR and a multi-investigator program project grant on milk allergy. Young investigators typically regard a robust portfolio of investigator-initiated research as a sign that a field will enjoy continued NIH support and, understandably, consider the level of that support in choosing career directions. Other challenges include the relatively narrow interests of the biotechnology and pharmaceutical industries in food allergy research compared to other immune-mediated diseases. For example, a survey of the federal clinical trials database (www.clinicaltrials.gov) revealed only six therapeutic intervention trials, two of which are sponsored by industry. Fortunately, recent advances may make the field more attractive to academic investigators and industry. These include the development of new and improved animal models and an evolving understanding of the molecular mechanisms involved in food allergy and anaphylaxis. These advances should enable the identification of new therapeutic targets and their preclinical evaluation.

Food allergy research has also benefited from the generous support of philanthropic organizations and advocacy groups. This support has been instrumental in establishing a number of university-based food allergy research programs and greatly enhanced the capabilities of the academic research community to conduct research sponsored, in part, by NIH.


## Basic and Preclinical Research

**Food allergens and their interactions with the immune system**. The majority of well-characterized inhalant and food allergens are water-soluble proteins. However, recent studies indicate that lipids and lipid-carbohydrate complexes (e.g., glycolipids extracted from cypress pollens) can trigger immune and allergic responses. While lipid food allergens have not yet been identified, new studies have revealed the molecular pathways by which lipid and glycolipids can activate the immune system.

Cells that express the surface marker CD4 constitute a common subset of the T lymphocytes, known as T helper cells, that circulate in the blood. Recent observations suggest that approximately 60 percent of the lung CD4+ cells in patients with moderate-to-severe persistent asthma may be not conventional CD4+ T helper cells, but a special type of lymphocyte, called a natural killer T (NKT) cell.[1] NKT cells are involved in the immune response to infectious agents and have been shown in mouse models to be involved in the development of asthma. NKT cells constitute a very rare population of circulating T cells and are activated by a special set of proteins (CD1d) on the surface of the antigen-presenting cells that display lipids and glycolipids to the immune system. These observations, plus the association of food allergy and asthma, suggest that glycolipid allergens and NKT cells may be involved in other allergic diseases, including food allergy.

Recent advances have also strengthened our understanding of the structure of protein allergens and how they interact with IgE antibodies. Protein structures can now be widely studied through advanced technologies, such as X-ray crystallography and nuclear magnetic resonance, which are capable of revealing three-dimensional structures and protein-protein interactions at the atomic level. Structural information can then be exploited to identify therapeutic targets and design novel drugs. Such structure-based insights may also be important for understanding the interactions between food allergens and the IgE antibodies to food. These antibodies recognize structures, called epitopes, within food allergens that can be of two different types: linear epitopes and conformational epitopes. How the immune system perceives these distinct epitopes appears to be important in food allergy. Individuals with persistent allergy to milk, egg, and peanut have IgE antibodies that recognize mainly linear epitopes, whereas those with transient allergy recognize a higher proportion of conformational epitopes. Analysis of epitope selection may eventually allow useful predictions about the future course of food allergy in individual subjects and provide the insights for novel therapeutic approaches.

Other studies indicate that subjects with a history of severe peanut allergy have IgE antibodies that recognize a broader range and larger number of distinct epitopes than those with less severe reactions. This greater IgE diversity correlates with higher levels of peanut allergen-triggered release of inflammatory mediators from basophils, a type of white blood cell involved in allergic inflammation.

**Animal models of food allergy and gastrointestinal immunity**. In the past, there were few mouse models of food allergy because it is difficu Animal models of food allergy and gastrointestinal immunity. In It to induce IgE antibody by oral administration of allergen. Within the last several years, NIAID-supported investigators have developed and characterized mouse models of human food allergy and related syndromes, such as eosinophilic gastroenteritis. Although rodent models of food allergy do not mimic all the features of human food allergy, some of the newer models display important characteristics of the human disease. As such, they should be useful for preclinical evaluation of new treatment and prevention strategies, and to define molecular and cellular mechanisms that may lead to new directions in food allergy research.

Studies of gastrointestinal immunity have demonstrated that the normal response to foods is oral tolerance, a state of immunological unresponsiveness that is established and maintained by a complex relationship between microbial flora in the gut and the immune cells of the gut mucosa. An emerging concept is that gut microbes and their products activate cells of the innate immune system, generating signals that strongly inhibit the development of allergic responses to foods. These inhibitory signals serve to maintain oral tolerance.

The availability of more informative animal models will undoubtedly facilitate high quality research that cannot be performed in humans; this research includes studies of exposure routes, mechanisms of the gut immune response, and the role of the mucosal barrier in the induction, maintenance, and loss of oral tolerance.

**Preclinical studies in animal models.** One immunotherapy approach being studied in mouse and larger animal models is to use a chimeric fusion protein, composed of part of another class of human antibody, IgG, fused to the major cat allergen, Fel d1. This and related constructs were developed based on recent insights regarding signaling pathways that down-regulate IgE-mediated responses. This approach was effective in blocking skin and systemic reactivity to Fel d1 when administered to humanized mice.

Another approach in a mouse model is to use bacteria engineered to produce recombinant and modified peanut proteins. The peanut proteins are modified so that they are less likely to induce allergic reactions. These bacteria are then heat-killed, after which they are administered rectally to mice. This experimental treatment modified the mouse immune response and protected peanut allergic mice from allergic reactions to peanut.

## Epidemiology and Genetics of Food Allergy and Anaphylaxis

**Epidemiology of food allergy and asthma.** Asthma is a risk factor for severe allergic reactions to foods, but only limited epidemiologic data address the relationship between asthma and food allergy. Similarly, we have few insights regarding the prevalence and incidence of food allergy in genetically or demographically defined population groups. One intriguing observation concerns children living in our nation's urban areas—a group known to have a high prevalence of asthma and high morbidity from asthma, but widely thought to have a relatively low incidence of certain immunologic diseases, including food allergy. However, a recent retrospective analysis, which was made possible through access to clinical samples obtained in the 1990s as a part of the NIAID-sponsored National Cooperative Inner-City Asthma Study, is shedding new light on this question. This analysis suggests that food allergy may, in fact, be a major co-morbid condition among inner-city children with asthma, in that about half of such subjects had detectable IgE antibodies to foods. Thus, food allergen sensitization is prevalent in inner-city children with asthma and appears to be associated with both increased hospitalization and a requirement for steroid treatment.

**Epidemiology of systemic food allergic reactions: mild and moderate vs. severe reactions.** Few studies have addressed predictive factors for severe reactions, but some limited clinical data are available. Individuals who require only a low dose of food to trigger food allergic responses (i.e., a low threshold) have an increased risk of severe systemic reactions to that food. However, the precise biological responses that determine these thresholds are not yet known. While higher levels of IgE antibodies to food predict the likelihood of an allergic reaction upon exposure to that food, the IgE antibody levels do not predict reaction severity.

A number of recent studies are providing intriguing insights into correlates of clinical severity that, if confirmed, may eventually serve as clinically useful biomarkers, or indicators, of food allergy severity. As previously mentioned, the number of allergen epitopes recognized by an individual may predict the severity of food-allergic reactions. Another recent study suggests that blood levels of an enzyme called platelet activating factor acetylhydrolase (PAF-AH) may be reduced in subjects with anaphylactic reactions to peanut as compared to healthy subjects and to children with non-fatal severe reactions to peanut. Further studies will be needed to determine the reproducibility of this finding and to discover whether comparable defects also increase the risk of anaphylaxis.

**Genetics of food allergy.** Recent advances, including the completion of the Human Genome Project (http://www.ornl. gov/sci/techre sources/Human_ Genome/home.shtml) and the HapMap project (http://www.hapmap.org/), a multi-country effort to identify and catalog genetic similarities and differences in human beings, are creating opportunities to define the genetics of human food allergy. A recent example of a link between genetic variability and allergic disorders concerns filaggrin, a protein that maintains skin and mucosal barrier function. Atopic dermatitis and asthma are strongly associated with a loss of function in the filaggrin gene. Currently, the relationship of filaggrin to food allergy, if any, is unknown. In other studies, a subset of children of Japanese descent diagnosed with atopic dermatitis and food allergy was shown to have a variant of the gene that codes for the serine protease inhibitor Krazal type 5 (SPINK5). Similar to the situation with filaggrin, SPINK5 contributes to the maintenance of the skin barrier.

**Epidemiology of eosinophilic esophagitis.** Eosinophilic esophagitis is an emerging disease, with an incidence of about one in 10,000 children per year. It has a high rate of association with atopic diseases (70 percent), including food allergy (46 percent). Genomic analysis from esophageal biopsies demonstrates markedly increased expression of a set of genes involved in eosinophil biology, especially the gene for eotaxin-3, a molecule that attracts eosinophils to sites of inflammation. Not only is there striking expression of eotaxin, but also a possible genetic link to disease susceptibility associated with a single nucleotide polymorphism (SNP) in the eotaxin gene.

## Clinical Trials to Prevent and Treat Food Allergy

**Prevention studies.** Recent observations support the conclusion that a number of novel approaches could be explored in food allergy prevention studies. A European study suggests that, in children with allergic rhinitis, immunotherapy with airborne allergens can prevent or delay the onset of asthma, but comparable studies have not been conducted in the area of food allergy. Another study showed that high levels of exposure to dog and cat allergens in early childhood reduces the development of allergy. This effect may be mediated by the dog and cat allergens themselves, or by microbial products, such as endotoxins, which are carried by pets and farm animals. Endotoxins are potent activators of innate immune responses that can skew immune responses away from the development of allergies. Thus, according to an emerging concept called the hygiene hypothesis, high levels of exposure to pets and farm animals results in exposure to microbial products, including endotoxins, and may condition the developing immune system toward a non-allergic state.

Other epidemiologic studies have reported that early life exposure to peanut is associated with remarkably low rates of peanut allergy. For example, more than 90 percent of Israeli children eat a popular peanut snack beginning in the first year of life. In contrast, young children in the United States, Europe, and Australia generally avoid peanuts or consume relatively small amounts. The prevalence of peanut allergy in Israel is 0.04 percent, roughly 10–20 fold lower than is observed in the United States, Europe, and Australia. Independent observations suggest that the immunological and clinical response to peanut allergens may also depend on cooking and preparation methods; roasting peanuts at high temperatures appears to alter the structure of allergens, possibly making them more allergenic.

Taken together, these findings suggest that early-life, high-dose allergen exposure might prevent the development of IgE antibody to that allergen. These possibilities are further borne out by experiments in rodents showing that oral or other mucosal exposure to allergen stimulates oral tolerance, particularly in neonatal rodents.

Currently, NIAID supports two clinical trials and associated mechanistic studies of early-life allergen exposure and its effects on the development of allergic diseases, including food allergy. In the first trial, which is focused specifically on a food allergen, peanut avoidance will be compared to daily oral peanut consumption, including the peanut snack popular with Israeli children. The study will determine whether this treatment prevents the development of peanut allergy in children from four to ten months of age. In the second trial, daily oral mucosal immunotherapy with grass, cat and house dust mite allergens will be provided for one year to children aged 18–30 months. These children will be assessed for the development of allergy to the test allergens, to other allergens including food allergens, and to the development of seasonal and perennial rhinitis and asthma.

**Treatment studies.** Several clinical studies have demonstrated the feasibility of immune-based approaches to treat food allergy, and further studies are in early planning stages. One approach has been to lower IgE antibody levels and the number of their receptors on mast cells and basophils through the use of monoclonal antibodies that bind to human IgE (anti-IgE antibodies). One such monoclonal antibody, omalizumab, was recently licensed by the U.S. Food and Drug Administration (FDA) for treatment of asthma. In one study, patients with peanut allergy were grouped according to their sensitivity to oral food challenge with peanut and then randomly assigned to either receive a placebo or graded doses of a monoclonal anti-IgE antibody that is believed to be similar to the FDA-approved drug. High doses of the monoclonal antibody raised the threshold for an allergic reaction to oral peanut challenge from about one half of a peanut to nine peanuts, a change generally believed to be clinically relevant. These results represent the clearest evidence that immune-based approaches have potential value in the management of severe food allergy, even if only to reduce the severity of reactions to an accidental exposure. However, additional evaluation of this therapy will be needed, as a subset of the subjects did not increase their threshold in response to treatment with anti-IgE antibodies.

In contrast to subcutaneous immunotherapy with airborne and insect venom allergens, subcutaneous injection of food allergens is associated with unacceptably high rates of severe allergic reactions. Hence, additional approaches are being devised to allow food allergen immunotherapy trials to proceed. These include allergen administration via the mucosal, rather than the subcutaneous, route; chemical modification or recombinant genetic engineering to modify allergen structures; use of peptide fragments rather than the intact protein allergen; and conduct of allergen immunotherapy studies under a protective umbrella provided by anti-IgE monoclonal antibody. In support of the latter approach, a recent study sponsored by NIAID and an industry partner showed that pre-treating adults with ragweed allergic rhinitis with the FDA-approved monoclonal anti-IgE antibody allowed them to undergo rush immunotherapy (a type of immunotherapy that involves a rapid increase in the dose of ragweed over a period of hours) with a five-fold lower risk of anaphylaxis to the ragweed allergen injections.

In another NIAID/industry partnership, ragweed allergen was chemically coupled to small immunostimulatory pieces of bacterial DNA that activate a component of the innate immune system. This conjugate was given subcutaneously to adults with ragweed allergies prior to the onset of ragweed season. In comparison to the placebo group, conjugate-treated subjects showed markedly reduced symptoms, an improvement that persisted through the following ragweed season, one year after therapy was discontinued.

If its safety and efficacy can be confirmed, such an approach could be adapted to food allergens.

As noted, one promising approach is to administer allergens by the mucosal route because mucosal delivery of allergens apparently induces a protective immune response with a markedly reduced risk of systemic allergic reactions. Tests of the mucosal route include the rectal administration, in mice, of the mutated peanut proteins mentioned above. To date, human trials have used oral therapy or sublingual immunotherapy (SLIT). SLIT in humans is associated with a substantially reduced risk of provoking serious adverse events after allergen administration. SLIT reduces symptoms of allergic rhinitis and, apparently, asthma. The mechanisms by which SLIT reduces allergic symptoms are unknown, but this approach has been used successfully in Europe and is undergoing trials in the United States. One trial has demonstrated that SLIT can be safe and effective in treating patients with hazelnut allergy.

Other studies are exploring allergen non-specific therapies, namely probiotics and Chinese herbal medicines. Probiotics are live microorganisms, such as *Lactobacillus* species, that may beneficially affect the host by improving the balance of intestinal microbes. Probiotics are present in fermented foods such as yogurt. Limited experimental data suggest that probiotics administered early in life to infants at high risk of developing allergic diseases may prevent or delay the onset of atopic dermatitis. In mouse models, probiotics may dampen certain immune-mediated inflammatory diseases, including experimental colitis. The underlying mechanisms are unclear, but may involve direct stimulation of the innate immune response and/or suppression of an adaptive allergic immune response. In mouse models, Chinese herbal medicines block peanut-induced anaphylaxis, even several weeks after therapy is discontinued. The mechanisms by which this occurs are not fully understood. Neither probiotics nor Chinese herbal medicines have been tested in human trials to prevent or treat food allergy.

**Impediments to clinical trials.** The Panel identified several current impediments to the conduct of clinical trials for food allergy. These include: 1) safety concerns related to the potential for severe adverse reactions associated with therapies that contain food allergens; 2) the need to study pediatric populations, as the allergens of interest, the immunologic mechanisms underlying disease, and severity of disease may differ in children and adults; 3) the need to study infants and young children in food allergy prevention trials; and 4) a lack of regulatory guidance on acceptable study designs.

Concerning the last point, the panel discussed two proposed general study designs and outcome measures.

In the first type of study, researchers would evaluate safety and efficacy of candidate drugs in the setting of double-blind, placebo-controlled food challenge (DBPCFC), the only method which allows assessment of the safety of a patient consuming a particular food under conditions where risks can be minimized. This study design includes observation under carefully monitored conditions and medical supervision, but involves risks associated with the food challenges. Even at experienced food allergy research centers, approximately 25 percent of DBPCFCs are associated with moderately severe reactions. Because of the risks inherent in DBPCFCs, the procedure is performed only by experienced investigators, who monitor subjects carefully during and after the food challenge and undertake early, definitive treatment of allergic reactions. These measures limit the severity of the reactions. Under these controlled conditions, epinephrine is used in approximately 10 percent of subjects with allergic reactions; there have been no fatal reactions in more than 5,000 oral food challenges performed by the experienced investigators in the NIAID Consortium of Food Allergy Research.

The second study design would assess safety and efficacy of drug vs. placebo in decreasing the frequency and severity of adverse reactions to accidental food allergen exposure. The latter study design eliminates the risks of DBPCFC, but requires large numbers of subjects to be followed for relatively long times. This study design also introduces confounding factors related to the lack of a controlled or documented exposure history and management of adverse events by physicians and emergency medical technicians not directly involved in the study. It is possible that each study design may have an appropriate role at different stages of drug development and licensure.

## Recommendations

The Expert Panel organized its recommendations into five areas: 1) Clinical Trials Design; 2) Clinical Trials to Prevent and Treat Food Allergy; 3) Epidemiology and Genetics of Food Allergy; 4) Basic and Pre-Clinical Research Studies; and 5) Research Resources. These are addressed in the following sections, giving priority to those areas believed to be most essential to future progress.

## Clinical Trials Design

The Panel recommends that the Secretary of Health and Human Services direct the NIH and the FDA to resolve impediments to the design and conduct of clinical trials for the prevention and treatment of food allergy. The Panel recommends that the agencies establish regular meetings as a mechanism to identify the critical issues and develop solutions, and submit a written update to the agency heads on progress at the end of one year. The Panel identified the following issues that need formal or informal FDA guidance in order to facilitate the design of food allergy clinical trials, accelerate progress in this area, and encourage additional research sponsors:

- Inclusion of pediatric subjects in clinical trials of food allergy treatment and prevention strategies
- Inclusion of subjects with history of anaphylaxis to food
- Use of DBPCFC in clinical research and clinical trials, including acceptable safety and efficacy endpoints for phase 2 and 3 DBPCFC trials; strengths and limitations of this approach; and appropriate allergen doses and dose escalations in DBPCFC studies
- Use of outcome of natural (accidental) exposure to food allergens as an efficacy endpoint for licensure studies; consideration of alternative study designs that can be conducted in a more controlled environment, such as DBPCFC
- Use of available biomarkers as risk stratification tools

Identification of the regulatory requirements, if any, for studies that use foods or food components as therapeutic agents

## Clinical Trials to Prevent and Treat Food Allergy

The Expert Panel recommends that the Secretary of Health and Human Services direct the NIH to evaluate promising new approaches in the prevention and treatment of food allergies in clinical studies and clinical trials. Promising approaches may include, but not be limited to:

## Prevention

- Treatment of high-risk, young children with high dose allergen by mucosal routes to prevent the development of food allergy
- Evaluation of the results of these trials to consider changing current guidelines on allergen avoidance in early childhood
- Assessment of probiotics as prevention measures

## Treatment

- Treatment with allergens in combination with agents that improve the safety of allergen immunotherapy
- Treatment with allergens modified to maintain immune responses but improve safety
- Treatment with allergens by routes of delivery different from subcutaneous (e.g., oral, nasal, sublingual, rectal)
- Treatment with a combination of approaches
- Assessment of non-allergen specific approaches

## Prevention and Treatment of Severe Food Allergic Reactions or Food-Induced Anaphylaxis

- Refinement of existing treatment protocols of severe reactions (e.g., intramuscular vs. subcutaneous epinephrine, early treatment with beta-adrenergic agonists, steroids, use of non-sedating antihistamines in infants)
- Use of pharmacological and immunological approaches to develop new therapies to prevent or more effectively treat severe reactions

## Interventions to Treat Eosinophil-Associated Mucosal Syndromes

- Development of therapies for this spectrum of diseases
- Definition of its relationship to food allergy

## Epidemiology And Genetics of Food Allergy

The Expert Panel recommends that the Secretary of Health and Human Services direct the NIH to investigate epidemiological, genetic, developmental, environmental and pathogenetic relationships between:

- Mild to moderately severe food-induced allergic reactions and severe, life-threatening reactions
- Reactions occurring only at high threshold doses of food exposure and those occurring at low threshold doses
- Atopic dermatitis and food allergy
- Asthma and food allergy
- Food allergy and eosinophilic gastrointestinal disorders

Epidemiologic and genetics studies may include, but not be limited to:

- Investigation of biomarkers of severe food allergy, foods associated with reaction severity, and genetic components of reaction severity
- Evaluation of the genetic basis of food allergy and whether it is distinct from genetic susceptibility to atopic dermatitis, asthma and allergic rhinitis
- Investigation of the relationship between mutations in the filaggrin gene and other candidate genes known to be associated with atopic dermatitis, and cutaneous sensitization to food allergens
- Investigation of the role of NKT cells, proposed as a marker of asthma, in food allergy

## Basic and Pre-Clinical Research Studies

The Expert Panel recommends that the Secretary of Health and Human Services direct the NIH to facilitate and promote investigator-initiated and solicited research on:

### *Allergen Structure*

- Evaluation of epitopes and their diversity in subsets of food allergic subjects
- Identification of new food allergens, especially non-aqueous allergens and post-translationally modified proteins

*Animal Models*

- Expansion of studies of genetic, environmental (e.g., microbial flora), and developmental factors that modulate sensitization vs. tolerance to food.
- Evaluation of mechanisms (immunological, mucosal barrier function, leukocyte trafficking) that mediate local immune responses
- Evaluation of biomarkers in animals that may be useful in assessing the occurrence, severity and resolution of severe responses/anaphylaxis to food in humans

## Research Resources

The Expert Panel recommends that the Secretary of Health and Human Services direct the NIH to determine the feasibility and utility of a national and international registry of food-induced allergic reactions, including the use of existing datasets; expansion of asthma studies to include these data; and opportunity costs.

- Development of a national/international database of food-induced allergic reactions, both after accidental exposure and in association with oral food challenges, and promotion of its use in epidemiologic and genetic studies and to facilitate clinical study design.

# APPENDIX A

## Expert Panel Members

**Rob C. Aalberse, Ph.D.**
University of Amsterdam
Amsterdam, Netherlands

**Kathleen Barnes, Ph.D.**
Johns Hopkins University School of Medicine
Baltimore, MD

**Stephen J. Galli, M.D. (Co-chair)**
Stanford University School of Medicine
Stanford, CA

**Raif S. Geha, M.D.**
The Children's Hospital
Boston, MA

**Susan L. Hefle, Ph.D.**[*]
University of Nebraska Department of Food Science and Technology
Lincoln, NE

**Patrick G. Holt, Ph.D., D.Sc., F.R.C.Path.**
Telethon Institute for Child Health Research
Subiaco, Australia

**Marc Jenkins, Ph.D.**
University of Minnesota School of Medicine
Minneapolis, MN

**Jean-Pierre Kinet, M.D.**
Beth Israel Deaconess Medical Center, Harvard Institutes of Medicine
Boston, MA
**Gideon Lack, M.D.**
Evelina Children's Hospital, St Thomas' Hospital
London, United Kingdom

**Mark Larché, Ph.D.**
Imperial College Faculty of Medicine
London, United Kingdom

**Donald Leung, M.D, Ph.D.**
National Jewish Medical and Research Center
Denver, CO

---

[*] Deceased

**Lloyd Mayer, M.D.**
Mount Sinai School of Medicine
New York, NY

**Dean D. Metcalfe, M.D. (Co-chair)**
National Institute of Allergy and Infectious Diseases,
NIH Bethesda, MD

**Cathryn R. Nagler-Anderson, Ph.D.**
Massachusetts General Hospital
Charlestown, MA

**Carole Ober, Ph.D.**
The University of Chicago
Chicago, IL

**Marc Rothenberg, M.D, PhD.**
University of Cincinnati College of Medicine
Cincinnati, OH

**Hugh Sampson, M.D.**
Mount Sinai School of Medicine,
New York, NY

**Scott H. Sicherer, M.D.**
Mount Sinai Hospital, Box 1198
New York, NY
**Gary A. Van Nest, Ph.D.**
Dynavax Technologies Corporation
Berkeley, CA

## Panel Observers

**Amal Assa'ad, M.D.**
Cincinnati Children's Hospital Medical Center
Cincinnati, OH

American College of Allergy, Asthma & Immunology (ACAAI) Representative

**Mr. David Bunning**
President, Bunning Food Allergy Foundation
Lake Forest, IL

**Mr. Mo Mayrides**
Asthma and Allergy Foundation of America (AAFA)
Washington, DC

**Ms. Anne Munoz-Furlong**
The Food Allergy & Anaphylaxis Network (FAAN)
Fairfax, VA

**Ms. Catherine Nnoka**
International Life Sciences Institute
Washington, DC

**Mr. Robert M. Pacenza**
Food Allergy Initiative New York, NY

**Thomas A.E. Platts-Mills, M.D., Ph.D.**
University of Virginia Medical Center
Charlottesville, VA
American Academy of Allergy Asthma & Immunology (AAAAI) Representative

**Mary Jane Selgrade, Ph.D.**
Environmental Protection Agency
Research Triangle Park, NC

**Barbara A. Solan, R.N.**
Member of the public
Saline, MI

**Howard Sosin, Ph.D.**
Founder, Clarissa Sosin Foundation
Fairfield, CT

**Joseph F. Urban, Ph.D.**
United States Department of Agriculture
Beltsville, MD

## NIAID, NIH, and HHS Staff

**Ms. Carole Cole**
National Institute of Allergy and Infectious Diseases, NIH
Bethesda, MD

**Gang Dong, M.D., Ph.D.**
National Institute of Allergy and Infectious Diseases, NIH
Bethesda, MD

**Matthew Fenton, Ph.D.**
National Institute of Allergy and Infectious Diseases, NIH
Bethesda, MD

**Ms. Michelle M. Grifka**
National Institute of Allergy and Infectious Diseases, NIH
Bethesda, MD

**Charles Hackett, Ph.D.**
National Institute of Allergy and Infectious Diseases, NIH
Bethesda, MD

**Travis Hauguel, M.S.**
National Institute of Allergy and Infectious Diseases, NIH
Bethesda, MD

**Stephen James, M.D.**
National Institute of Diabetes and Digestive and Kidney Diseases, NIH
Bethesda, MD

**Joy Laurienzo, R.N.**
National Institute of Allergy and Infectious Diseases, NIH
Bethesda, MD

**Stefano Luccioli, M.D.**
Office of Food Additive Safety, CFSAN/Food and Drug Administration
College Park, MD

**Ms. Jean McKay, M.L.S.**
National Institute of Allergy and Infectious Diseases, NIH
Bethesda, MD

**James McNamara, M.D.**
National Institute of Allergy and Infectious Diseases, NIH
Bethesda, MD

**Michael Minnicozzi, Ph.D.**
National Institute of Allergy and Infectious Diseases, NIH
Bethesda, MD

**Marshall Plaut, M.D.**
National Institute of Allergy and Infectious Diseases, NIH
Bethesda, MD

**Lawrence Prograis, M.D.**
National Institute of Allergy and Infectious Diseases, NIH
Bethesda, MD

**Cristian Rodriguez, M.D.**
National Institute of Allergy and Infectious Diseases, NIH
Bethesda, MD

**Annette Rothermel, Ph.D.**
National Institute of Allergy and Infectious Diseases, NIH
Bethesda, MD

**Daniel Rotrosen, M.D.**
National Institute of Allergy and Infectious Diseases, NIH
Bethesda, MD

**Richard T. Sawyer, Ph.D.**
National Institute of Allergy and Infectious Diseases, NIH
Bethesda, MD

**Captain Ernestine Smartt, R.N.**
National Institute of Allergy and Infectious Diseases, NIH
Bethesda, MD

**Dana Smith, J.D.**
National Institute of Allergy and Infectious Diseases, NIH
Bethesda, MD

**Mary Smolskis, R.N.**
National Institute of Allergy and Infectious Diseases, NIH
Bethesda, MD

# APPENDIX B (AGENDA)

Bethesda North Marriott Hotel
5701 Marinelli Road
Rockville, Maryland 20852

## Monday, March 13, 2006

| | |
|---|---|
| 7:30 a.m. | **Arrival/Sign In**<br>Continental Breakfast |
| 8:00 a.m. | **Welcome, Purpose of this Meeting**<br>Daniel Rotrosen, M.D., Director, Division of Allergy,<br>Immunology and Transplantation, NIAID, NIH |
| 8:10 a.m. | **Introduction: Nature and Scope of the Problem**<br>Discussion Leaders: Stephen Galli, M.D., Stanford and<br>Dean Metcalfe, M.D., NIAID |
| 8:30 a.m. | **Review of NIH Food Allergy Portfolio**<br>Richard Sawyer, Ph.D., NIAID and Marshall Plaut,<br>M.D., NIAID |

| | |
|---|---|
| 9:00 a.m. | **Consortium of Food Allergy Research**<br>Hugh Sampson, M.D., Mount Sinai[*] |
| 9:30 a.m. | **Break** |
| 9:45 a.m. | **Allergen Structure and Its Implications for Bioengineered Foods**<br>Rudolf Valenta, M.D., University of Vienna[**] |
| 10:30 a.m. | **Pathogenesis and Thresholds**<br>Susan Hefle, Ph.D., University of Nebraska Lincoln |
| 11:15 a.m. | **Genetics of Food Allergy**<br>Carole Ober, Ph.D., University of Chicago |
| 12:00 p.m. | **New Therapeutic Approaches to Food Allergy**<br>Donald Leung, M.D., Ph.D., National Jewish Medical and Research Center |
| 12:45 p.m. | **WorkingLunch, discussion of breakout sessions**<br>Stephen Galli, M.D., Stanford and Dean Metcalfe, M.D., NIAID |
| 1:30 p.m. | **Breakout Sessions I**<br><br>**Severe Reactions and Anaphylaxis**<br>Gideon Lack, M.D., St. Mary's Hospital, chair; Stephen Galli, M.D., Stanford, co-chair; Lloyd Mayer, M.D., Mt. Sinai; Dean Metcalfe, M.D., NIAID.<br><br>**Antigen Structure**<br>Rob Aalberse, Ph.D., Sanquin Research, chair; Rudolf Valenta, M.D.[**], University of Vienna, co-chair; Jean- |

[*] Hugh Sampson, M.D., Mount Sinai, was unable to attend the Panel meeting on the first day. His presentation, "Consortium of Food Allergy Research," was made by Dr Scott Sicherer, Mount Sinai.

[**] Rudolf Valenta, M.D., University of Vienna was unable to attend the Panel meeting. His presentation, "Allergen Structure and Its Implications for Bioengineered Foods," was made by Dr. Dean Metcalfe, NIAID, NIH.

Pierre Kinet, M.D., Beth Israel Hospital; Cathryn Nagler-Anderson, Ph.D., Massachusetts General Hospital.

**Atopic Dermatitis**
Raif Geha, M.D., Ph.D., Children's Hospital Boston, chair; Donald Leung, M.D., Ph.D., National Jewish, co-chair; Hugh Sampson, M.D.[*], Mt. Sinai; Mark Larche, Ph.D., Imperial College London.

**Genetics of Food Allergy**
Kathleen Barnes, Ph.D., Johns Hopkins University, chair; Carole Ober, Ph.D., University of Chicago co-chair; Marc Rothenberg, M.D., Ph.D., University of Cincinnati; Gary Van Nest, Ph.D., Dynavax.

**Thresholds**
Scott Sicherer, M.D., Mount Sinai chair; Susan Hefle, Ph.D., University of Nebraska Lincoln co-chair; Patrick Holt, Ph.D., University of Western Australia; Marc Jenkins, Ph.D., University of Minnesota.

3:00 p.m. **Break**

3:45 p.m. **Review of Breakout Sessions I and Recommendations**
Discussion Leaders: Stephen Galli, M.D., Stanford and Dean Metcalfe, M.D., NIAID, NIH.

5:15 p.m. **Adjourn**

6:30 p.m. **Dinner**
Tragara (Restaurant)
4935 Cordell Avenue

---

[**] Rudolf Valenta, M.D., University of Vienna was unable to attend the Panel meeting. His presentation, "Allergen Structure and Its Implications for Bioengineered Foods," was made by Dr. Dean Metcalfe, NIAID, NIH.

[*] Hugh Sampson, M.D., Mount Sinai, was unable to attend the Panel meeting on the first day. His presentation, "Consortium of Food Allergy Research," was made by Dr Scott Sicherer, Mount Sinai.

Bethesda, MD 20814

# Tuesday, March 14, 2006

7:30 a.m.          **Arrival/Sign In**
                   Continental Breakfast

8:00 a.m.          **Breakout Sessions II**

                   **Animal Models of Food Allergy**
                   athryn Nagler-Anderson, PhD. Mass General, chair;
                   Raif Geha, M.D., Children's Hospital, co-chair; Stephen
                   Galli, M.D., Stanford; Susan Hefle, Ph.D., University of
                   Nebraska.

                   **Eosinophils and Mucosal Syndromes**
                   Marc Rothenberg, M.D., Ph.D., Children's Hospital,
                   Cincinnati, chair; Lloyd Mayer, M.D., Mount Sinai, co-
                   chair; Rob Aalberse, Ph.D., Sanquin Research; Dean
                   Metcalfe, M.D., NIAID.

                   **Novel Therapeutic Approaches**
                   Jean-Pierre Kinet, M.D., Beth Israel Boston, chair; Gary
                   Van Nest, Ph.D., Dynavax, Co-chair; Donald Leung,
                   M.D., Ph.D., National Jewish; Carole Ober, Ph.D.,
                   University of Chicago.

                   **Respiratory Allergy and Food Allergy**
                   Mark Larche, Ph.D., Imperial College London, chair;
                   Hugh Sampson, M.D., Mount Sinai, co-chair; Kathleen
                   Barnes, Ph.D., Johns Hopkins University; Scott
                   Sicherer, M.D.; Mount Sinai.

                   **Tolerance and Food Allergy**
                   Patrick Holt, Ph.D., University of Western Australia,
                   chair; Marc Jenkins, Ph.D., University of Minnesota,

co-chair; Gideon Lack, M.D., St. Mary's Hospital; Rudolf Valenta, M.D.[**], University of Vienna.

| | |
|---|---|
| 9:30 a.m. | **Break** |
| 9:45 a.m. | **Comments from the Audience** |
| 10:30 p.m. | **Review of Breakout Session II and Recommendations**<br>Discussion Leaders: Stephen Galli, M.D., Stanford and Dean Metcalfe, M.D., NIAID |
| 12:45 p.m. | **WorkingLunch, final summary discussion** |
| 1:15 p.m. | **Adjourn** |

# End Notes

[1] After the Food Allergy Expert Panel report was completed, further data were published indicating that NKT cells are not increased in asthma and that these cells represent less than 1% of the lung CD4+ cells. Other published studies demonstrated significant increases in NKT cells in subjects with moderate to severe asthma, but the total number of NKT cells was less than 1% of the lung CD4+ cells. Despite these differing observations, the role of NKT cells in allergic diseases, including food allergy, merits further investigation.

---

[**] Rudolf Valenta, M.D., University of Vienna was unable to attend the Panel meeting. His presentation, "Allergen Structure and Its Implications for Bioengineered Foods," was made by Dr. Dean Metcalfe, NIAID, NIH.

In: Food Allergy Overview and Children's...        ISBN: 978-1-61728-478-6
Editor: Lee R. Daniels                    © 2010 Nova Science Publishers, Inc.

*Chapter 6*

# THE ROLE OF NIH BIOMEDICAL RESEARCH IN ADDRESSING FOOD ALLERGY[*]

## *Anthony S. Fauci*

National Institute of Allergy and Infectious Diseases

Mr. Chairman and members of the Subcommittee, thank you for the opportunity to discuss with you today food allergy and the research being conducted and supported by the National Institutes of Health (NIH) to address this public health problem. Within NIH, the National Institute of Allergy and Infectious Diseases (NIAID) is the lead institute for research in this area, although other NIH Institutes and Centers support basic research relevant to food allergy. I am particularly pleased to be here with you as we recognize the 11th Annual Food Allergy Awareness Week and commend your efforts to bring attention to this important issue.

## OVERVIEW OF FOOD ALLERGY

Food allergy is much more than an inconvenience; the effects of food allergy can be devastating and sometimes deadly for those afflicted. During an

---

[*] This is an edited, reformatted and augmented version of a statement dated May 2008.

allergic response to food, the immune system overreacts to certain components of foods, setting off a cascade of immunological events that leads to symptoms ranging from itchy hives to anaphylaxis. Anaphylaxis is a severe and life-threatening systemic allergic reaction characterized by fall of blood pressure, upper airway obstruction, and difficulty breathing. Food allergy causes an estimated 30,000 episodes of anaphylaxis each year, accounting for approximately one-third to one-half of all anaphylaxis-related emergency room visits. Food allergy also causes an estimated 100 to 200 deaths per year in the United States. It is truly sobering to consider that, as a consequence of food allergies, two or three otherwise healthy Americans – usually adolescents or young adults – may lose their lives this week. Even with diligent avoidance of known food allergens, it is estimated that each year, one of every four food-allergic individuals will have an accidental exposure that leads to a food-induced allergic reaction.

Food allergies affect approximately 6 to 8 percent of children under four years of age and about 4 percent of adults in the United States. Evidence suggests that the prevalence of food allergy is increasing, especially peanut allergies, which tend to persist throughout life. Severe, life-threatening reactions occur mostly in adolescents and young adults, and peanuts and tree nuts are the most common causes of such reactions. Currently, the only proven interventions for food allergy are allergen avoidance and treatment with antihistamines, and intravenous fluids and epinephrine for more severe reactions.

Food allergy affects the health, nutrition, development, and quality of life of children and adults. Because a history of mild reactions does not preclude the occurrence of future life-threatening reactions, food allergies can also have disconcerting psychological effects related to fears of serious reactions and the stigma related to avoidance of common foods and social gatherings. As you are undoubtedly aware, this is a particular problem for children in school lunchrooms and other social settings where others may minimize or fail to understand the seriousness of the allergy. The increasing prevalence of certain food allergies, their persistence throughout life, the potential for fatal allergic reactions, and the lack of preventive approaches other than food avoidance have all contributed to the emergence of food allergy as an important public health problem.

## CURRENT NIAID RESEARCH ON FOOD ALLERGY

NIAID is the principal sponsor of food allergy research within the U.S. Government. This support has increased significantly over the last five years, from $1.2 million in fiscal year (FY) 2003 to an estimated $13.4 million in FY 2008, a greater than ten-fold increase. NIAID-supported food allergy research includes basic and preclinical research on the immune mechanisms involved in food allergy, research to understand the epidemiology and genetics of food allergy, and clinical studies to treat and prevent food allergy. Like all of NIH, NIAID awards grants to researchers whose investigator-initiated proposals are judged in peer review to be of high quality. NIAID also solicits research proposals through special initiatives that target particular areas of inquiry and foster collaboration within the field. These initiatives and networks include the NIAID Consortium of Food Allergy Research, the Asthma and Allergic Diseases Cooperative Research Centers, the Immune Tolerance Network, and the Inner City Asthma Consortium. NIAID also supports intramural investigators on our Bethesda, Maryland, campus who work on allergic diseases and anaphylaxis, including a new program focused specifically on food allergy.

In addition, NIAID supports a much larger portfolio of basic research on immunologic and allergic mechanisms that is relevant to the problem of food allergies. In FY 2007, support for this broader research portfolio totaled more than $500 million. The Institute's broad support of basic research in allergy and immunology provides a critical foundation that is advancing the field of food allergy, providing scientists with a better understanding of how the healthy immune system averts the development of allergy and of the mechanisms that contribute to allergy. Food allergy is frequently accompanied by other allergic diseases including atopic dermatitis (eczema) and asthma. The latter is an important risk factor for severe allergic reactions to food. Thus, research findings in the broader areas of immunology, including asthma and allergic diseases, likely will move the field of food allergy forward.

In the area of basic research in food allergy, researchers are studying the molecular structure of food allergens and their interactions with the immune system, including the immunoglobulin E (IgE) antibodies that mediate allergic reactions to food. For example, scientists are analyzing the specific structures, called epitopes, in food allergens that are recognized by IgE antibodies. These structures — and how they are recognized by the immune system — may determine the severity of a person's allergic responses and the persistence of allergy throughout his or her life. NIAID-supported scientists also are conducting basic research on the components of the immune system that play a role in anaphylaxis, studying the molecular events that precipitate and characterize anaphylactic reactions, and conducting long-term studies of patients with food allergies.

Preclinical studies include the development and characterization of animal models of food allergy. Improved mouse models, which have been developed in recent years by NIAID-supported researchers, mimic many of the important characteristics of human food allergy. Potential approaches to treating and preventing food allergy are being evaluated in such animal models, as a prelude to human studies. Some experimental approaches are relying on the use of allergenic foods as immunotherapeutics, capable of eliciting immunological tolerance with repeated, controlled administration. Other investigators are treating patients with structurally modified foods that are less likely to cause serious allergic reactions, but which may still elicit a state of tolerance. The safety of one such experimental treatment, the use of bacteria engineered to produce modified peanut proteins, may eventually be tested in non-allergic adult volunteers and, if proven safe, in allergic individuals.

Very little is known about why only certain people develop food allergies. Research on the epidemiology and genetics of food allergy may provide insight into the genesis of food allergy and suggest approaches that may preempt children from developing allergies to certain foods. For example, the NIAID-supported Consortium of Food Allergy Research is conducting an observational study in which more than 400 infants who have allergies to milk or eggs have been enrolled, most of whom will lose their allergies to milk and eggs within a few years. Some of these children will develop allergy to peanuts. The study will follow the children for at least five years and study immunologic changes that accompany either the loss of allergy to foods or the development of allergy to peanut. Another study, the Urban Environmental Factors and Childhood Asthma Study, a project of the Inner City Asthma Consortium, is an observational study monitoring a cohort of children from birth for a number of factors, including the appearance of specific IgE antibodies to foods. This study will provide epidemiological data to address the relationship between asthma and food allergy.

The results of basic, preclinical, and epidemiological research have suggested a number of approaches for the prevention and treatment of food allergy. These approaches are being evaluated in several current and planned clinical trials. For example, in the United States, until earlier this year, the pediatric medicine community generally recommended avoidance of exposure to peanuts and other common food allergens during early life. However, epidemiological studies have raised the possibility that early life exposure to peanuts may lower the rate of peanut allergy. More than 90 percent of Israeli children eat a popular peanut snack called Bamba starting before their first birthday, yet the prevalence of peanut allergy in Israel is 10- to 20-fold lower than in the United States. To test the hypothesis that early exposure may prevent food allergies, the NIAID-sponsored Immune Tolerance Network is conducting a trial to determine whether feeding a peanut-containing snack to young children at risk of developing peanut allergy will prevent its development.

With regard to treatment of established food allergies, a number of trials are ongoing or in the planning stages. The Consortium of Food Allergy Research is conducting or planning several pilot trials of oral and sublingual (under the tongue) immunotherapy in egg- and peanut-allergic subjects to study safety and the ability of these approaches to desensitize subjects with allergies and induce immunological tolerance to the test allergens. In addition, the NIAID Asthma and Allergic Diseases Cooperative Research Centers are developing a clinical trial to evaluate whether, in combination with oral milk, a currently licensed drug for allergic asthma can reduce the incidence and severity of adverse effects of milk immunotherapy and facilitate the development of tolerance in patients with milk allergy.

The field of food allergy research has benefited greatly from the support and involvement of advocacy groups and philanthropic organizations. Included among these are the Food Allergy and Anaphylaxis Network, the Food Allergy Initiative, and the Food Allergy Project, each of which supports public awareness efforts, scientific workshops, and/or research projects, either independently or in collaboration with NIH.

## FUTURE PLANS

In March 2006, as required by the Food Allergen and Consumer Protection Act of 2004 (Pub. L. 108-282), NIAID convened the NIH Expert Panel on Food Allergy Research. The Panel reviewed basic and clinical efforts related to food allergies and made recommendations to the Secretary of Health and Human Services for enhancing and coordinating research activities related to food allergies. The findings and recommendations of the Panel were summarized in a report released in June 2007 and available at http://www3.niaid.nih.gov/topics/foodAllergy/research/ReportFoodAllergy.ht m.

The Panel discussed the challenges that NIH faces in the area of food allergy research, including the need to expand the relatively small cadre of scientists working in this area. To address this concern, in August 2007, NIAID announced a research initiative, *Exploratory Investigations in Food Allergy*, that will support innovative pilot studies and developmental research on the mechanisms of food allergy, with a goal of attracting additional investigators to the field of food allergy research. We are particularly gratified that almost all of the applicants for this initiative are new to the field of food allergy research and that approximately one-third have not had prior NIH funding. Co-sponsors include the Food Allergy and Anaphylaxis Network, the Food Allergy Project, and the U.S. Environmental Protection Agency. NIAID expects to award grants under this initiative this month.

The Panel also identified a number of impediments, concerns, and challenges to the conduct of clinical trials for the prevention and treatment of food allergy. One such challenge is the difficulty of studying new approaches in pediatric patients, including infants. Other concerns relate to the potential for severe reactions to foods or food allergens in treatment or prevention trials and the current lack of tools to identify those at the highest risk for such reactions. The Panel recommended that Secretary of Health and Human Services direct the NIH and the Food and Drug Administration (FDA) to resolve impediments to the design and conduct of clinical trials for the prevention and treatment of food allergy. In response to this recommendation, NIH and FDA will convene a workshop next month on the design of food allergy clinical trials.

The Panel also made a number of recommendations regarding the future of food allergy research, including those related to clinical trials, epidemiology and genetics, basic and preclinical studies, and research resources. A number of the research activities described earlier address these recommendations. NIAID is firmly committed to implementing the remaining recommendations.

In addition to its research portfolio in food allergy, NIAID supports other activities to improve the lives of those who are affected by food allergy. For example, NIAID is coordinating the development of comprehensive clinical guidelines for the diagnosis and management of food allergy. This effort will provide guidance to clinicians, families, and patients for diagnosing and managing food allergies. NIAID will convene a Coordinating Committee in the summer of 2008 to oversee the drafting of these guidelines. The guidelines will be prepared through a two-pronged approach, including an independent evidence-based literature review and consensus opinion developed by an expert panel. More than 20 professional societies, advocacy groups, and NIH Institutes and Centers will be involved in this process.

## CONCLUSION

With evidence indicating an increasing prevalence of food allergy in the United States, food allergy and associated anaphylaxis have emerged as important public health problems, particularly in children. Over the last five years, NIAID has substantially increased its support for basic, clinical and epidemiological research on food allergy and anaphylaxis. While much progress has been made in the scientific understanding of food allergies and in the public's awareness of difficulties in managing them, many challenges remain. NIAID is strongly committed to the goal of reducing the burden of food allergy for the millions of affected children and their families in the United States by continuing and expanding support for research to understand food allergies, by bringing new scientists into this research area, and by developing interventions for treatment and prevention.

In: Food Allergy Overview and Children's...          ISBN: 978-1-61728-478-6
Editor: Lee R. Daniels                      © 2010 Nova Science Publishers, Inc.

*Chapter 7*

# STATEMENT OF TERESA WALTERS, BEFORE THE SENATE HEALTH, EDUCATION, LABOR AND PENSIONS COMMITTEE, HEARING ON "ADDRESSING THE CHALLENGE OF CHILDREN WITH FOOD ALLERGIES"*

## *Teresa Walters*

Chairman Dodd, Ranking Member Alexander and distinguished Members of the Committee, thank you for inviting me here today. It is also a pleasure to address this panel that contains my home state Senator from Colorado. This Committee is doing a great service to millions of families around the country who have children with life-threatening food allergies. I am especially appreciative of Senator Dodd's efforts to champion S. 1232 and provide greater resources for schools who are struggling daily with the challenges posed by food allergies.

You have already heard some information about childhood food allergies and the speakers that follow me will share their perspectives as doctors, nurses, teachers and parents of food allergic children. You have heard food allergies referred to as "life-threatening," and you may consider that overly

---

* This is an edited, reformatted and augmented version of a statement dated May 2008.

dramatic. After all, a lot of medical conditions can be life-threatening if they are not treated properly. But I am here today to share my perspective as a mother who found out first-hand what life-threatening means. Almost exactly seven years ago, my son Nathan died from a severe allergic reaction to peanuts. He was 9 years old.

Nathan's third grade class in Washington state was scheduled to go to a local farm, along with two additional third grade classes. By the time the bus got to the farm, it was close enough to lunchtime that the school lunches were passed out. Lunch consisted of a peanut butter and jelly sandwich, trail mix with peanuts and a peanut butter cookie. A special lunch was supposed to have been ordered for Nathan, but wasn't. He received the same lunch as the other kids.

When he realized what was in his sack lunch, he returned the sandwich and trail mix to his teacher and told him that he couldn't have those things, he was allergic to peanuts. His teacher commended his awareness and Nate returned to his friends, thinking that he could eat what looked like a sugar cookie. Nathan didn't realize that he was eating a peanut butter cookie and didn't recognize the taste. When he was about halfway through, he commented to his friends that his tummy felt funny and again alerted his teacher that he didn't feel well.

His teacher recruited the assistance of a parent volunteer, who was also a nurse practitioner to sit with Nate on the bus, so the other kids wouldn't have to miss out on their field trip. Nathan had with him his inhaler and an Epipen. Nathan sat on that bus for 2-3 hours. When the field trip was over, it was decided that a parent would drive Nathan home, rather than back to school. The nurse practitioner would go along.

Witnesses say that Nathan was unable to walk unassisted at this point and looked like elephant man. By this time, he had been given a few sips of sprite and his inhaler. He was lain down in the back seat and Nathan finally left the farm, approximately three hours after ingesting a few bites of a cookie. A few minutes into the drive, the nurse practitioner asked the parent driver if she thought it advisable to give Nathan his epipen. The other parent didn't know what that was, but knew that Nathan was in serious trouble and quickly pulled into a fire station a few miles away from the farm. Nathan had stopped breathing and his heart had stopped beating by now.

One of the women ran into the fire station and asked if oxygen was available. Most of the fire fighters were out of the station on training, but one of the volunteer fire fighters was there. He called 911, followed the woman to the car and he was the one who finally administered Nathan's Epipen. He also began CPR. Less than one minute later, paramedics arrived and took over life saving efforts while racing to the hospital. I'm told that the doctors worked on him for over an hour; past the point of hope.

My understanding is that Nathan might have survived if he had been given his Epipen, especially considering how close emergency medical care was. I *know* he would have survived if his health care plan had been followed; if his school had received additional training on the severity and risks of food allergies.

As I am sure you can imagine, the death of my son was simply devastating. It was a year before I could even think about going back to work, and not a day goes by that I don't think about him and wonder what he would be doing now if he were still here with me. I live in Colorado now and I re-married a year ago. Fifteen years after being adamant about not wanting to go through the terror of possibly having another child with severe food allergies, my husband and I recently found out some wonderful news. I am four months pregnant with our first child together. I am doing all the usual pregnancy things – eating right, taking care of myself, trying to get a lot of sleep. But no doctor can tell me what I can do to make sure that my daughter does not develop a severe food allergy like Nathan did. The doctors simply don't know why Nate had a food allergy and they can't tell us why so many more children are developing these life-threatening allergies every year.

I appreciate what this Committee is doing today to focus attention on the issue of life-threatening food allergies. This issue is not going away. There are a lot of important public policy issues facing this Congress and our nation. Focusing on childhood food allergies needs to move up on our priority list. I urge you to do what you can to make sure that no parent has to endure what Nathan's dad and I have. Congress has the power to increase research funding, to protect children in the school environment, and to raise public awareness so that food allergies are treated like the serious, life-threatening medical condition that they are. Much more needs to be done.

Thank you.

In: Food Allergy Overview and Children's...      ISBN: 978-1-61728-478-6
Editor: Lee R. Daniels                    © 2010 Nova Science Publishers, Inc.

*Chapter 8*

# TESTIMONY OF HUGH A. SAMPSON, CHIEF OF PEDIATRIC ALLERGY & IMMUNOLOGY, DIRECTOR OF THE JAFFE FOOD ALLERGY INSTITUTE, MOUNT SINAI SCHOOL OF MEDICINE, HEARING ON "ADDRESSING THE CHALLENGE OF CHILDREN WITH FOOD ALLERGIES"[*]

## *Hugh A. Sampson*

My name is Hugh Sampson, and I am pleased to be here today to participate in this important hearing on the challenges confronting food-allergic children and their families. I am the Chief of the Pediatric Allergy and Immunology Division and the Director of the Jaffe Food Allergy Institute at the Mount Sinai School of Medicine in New York. I have spent over 25 years conducting research and caring for children with food allergic disorders. I am also president of the American Academy of Allergy, Asthma, and Immunology (AAAAI), an international organization of over 6,500 allergist/

---

[*] This is an edited, reformatted and augmented version of a testimony dated May 2008.

immunologists, allied health professionals, and others with a special interest in the research and treatment of allergic diseases.

I would like to begin by thanking you, Senator Dodd, for holding this important hearing during *Food Allergy Awareness Week*. Families across America will be working this week to educate their communities about food allergies, and it is inspiring for them to know that you are doing the same here in the United States Senate. In addition, I am grateful for your leadership as the sponsor of S. 1232, the *Food Allergy and Anaphylaxis Management Act*, and for your support for Federal policies to protect food allergic-children. Passage of your legislation is critically important to the ability of schools and parents to assure the safety of children with food allergies.

In addition, I am pleased to have the opportunity to express the strong support of the AAAAI for the *"Five Steps Forward for Food Allergy"* initiative announced just yesterday by the Food Allergy and Anaphylaxis Network (FAAN), a national organization dedicated to raising public awareness of food allergies through education and advocacy. I serve as Medical Director of FAAN, and believe that if the five recommended policy initiatives are implemented, we *will* reduce the incidence of fatal food allergic reactions in our country.

## BACKGROUND ON FOOD ALLERGY

While I know you are well aware of the impact of food allergies, Senator Dodd, I would like to provide some general information for the benefit of the Committee members. A food allergy occurs when a person's immune system "attacks" harmless proteins in our food. The immune system is the part of the body that usually fights infections and other harmful substances, but in this case the responses are misdirected. A food is misidentified as the body's enemy, and the immune system "fights" the food as it would a parasite or infection.

In children, the most common foods causing significant reactions are milk, egg, peanuts, tree nuts, fish, shellfish, soy and wheat, while in adults the most common foods are shellfish, peanuts, tree nuts and fish. Most children outgrow their allergies to many foods, but not typically to peanuts, nuts, fish, and shellfish, which are often considered life-long allergies.

In the majority of food allergic reactions, the symptoms will begin within minutes after an exposure, although a delay of up to an hour or more is possible. Some reactions can be mild including itchy skin and rashes, itchy mouth, and stomach aches. The more severe and life-threatening anaphylactic reactions can include swelling, hives, welts or itchiness of the skin; digestive symptoms such as severe stomach pain, nausea, vomiting, and diarrhea; respiratory symptoms such as hoarseness, difficulty swallowing, trouble breathing, wheezing, repetitive coughing, and in the worst cases, throat closing; and reduced blood circulation resulting in paleness, dizziness, passing out, low blood pressure, and even loss of pulse. Sometimes a reaction will subside and then start up again 1 to 3 hours later. There are also a number of gastrointestinal allergies that come on more slowly but can lead to abdominal pain and nausea, weight loss and failure to thrive.

There is no cure for food allergy. Strict avoidance of the allergy-causing food is the only way to avoid a reaction, but even trace amounts of a food allergen invisible to the naked eye, such as residual food on dishes and utensils simply wiped clean, can cause a severe reaction. In some cases the food does not even have to be swallowed. Inhaled food proteins vaporized during cooking have caused severe and even fatal reactions in some individuals. Prompt administration of epinephrine, also called "adrenaline," is the best method we now have for controlling a severe reaction. It is available by prescription as a self-injectable device.

More than 10 million Americans have food allergies, including almost 3 million children. The prevalence is highest in young children, with 6-8 percent of children under four years of age affected by food allergies. The prevalence of food allergies and associated anaphylaxis is increasing. For example, in a national survey, we found that the rates of peanut allergy doubled in children less than 5 years of age from 1997 to 2002, and similar findings were reported in the U.K. Globally, food allergies are most prevalent in industrialized countries like ours with similar lifestyles and eating habits. Through research, we are trying to identify the causes of this dramatic increase. There are several theories under investigation including the question of whether children in our culture are exposed to fewer germs, thereby requiring the immune system to be less active in fighting germs and somehow making it less effective at identifying certain foods as harmless. The onset of food allergy is often preceded by atopic dermatitis, commonly known as eczema, in which the normal skin barrier is defective. Another theory suggests that contact with creams containing food proteins or residual food on the hands of parents, caregivers and siblings may sensitize these children to the food. Other theories include the rise in consumption of omega-6-containing foods and decreased consumption of omega-3 polyunsaturated fatty acid-containing foods, reduced dietary antioxidants, and excess or deficiency of vitamin D. The majority of young children with food allergies and atopic dermatitis go on to develop respiratory allergies and asthma, something allergists call the "allergic march." In addition, children with food allergies and asthma are more likely to suffer from severe asthma, and are at greatest risk for severe and occasionally fatal anaphylactic reactions. We believe that a better understanding of the inter-relationship of these diseases is critical to developing new methods to prevent and treat food allergies.

This gives you some idea of the challenges that food allergies present to health care professionals. The impact in the real world of children and families is far more difficult to describe. Food is at the center of almost all of our social functions, and therefore presents a potential threat to the food allergic individual everywhere he or she turns. As I found with my second daughter, who has allergy to walnuts, parents must spend hours in grocery stores scrutinizing labels and phoning companies to get clarification on ingredient labels. In addition, many parents of a child with food allergies live every day knowing their child can walk out the door to day care, or school, or church, or camp, or literally any place in which food is served and end that day in the emergency room, in the hospital, or in an intensive care unit on a ventilator, or rarely, even dead. Data from an FDA survey published in January of this year, utilizing the National Electronic Injury Surveillance System of selected emergency departments around the U.S., suggest that there are about 125,000 emergency room visits each year for food allergy, and that about 15,000 of these are for anaphylactic reactions, with over 3,000 ending in hospitalizations. Somewhat alarming was the fact that only 43% of the anaphylactic cases were accurately diagnosed by the emergency room staff, a finding frequently reported in similar surveys, emphasizing the need for better health education training and guidelines for health care professionals. Other surveys suggest even higher numbers of anaphylaxis cases, and while accurate data is very difficult to come by, it is estimated that anaphylaxis caused by food allergy results in 100-150 deaths each year in our country. Death can be sudden, sometimes occurring within minutes. You can imagine how the life of an entire family is completely disrupted as they strive to avoid this fate. Far worse, imagine seeing your daughter die in a shopping mall while you are out looking for her prom dress, or your young son go into shock and eventually die from tasting some of a peanut snack unbeknownst to you while your are watching the Super Bowl together, or learning that your son died on a camp canoe trip from an anaphylactic reaction due to residual peanut butter on a knife used to make his sandwich.

# RECOMMENDATIONS

As I noted earlier, the American Academy of Allergy, Asthma & Immunology and I, personally, strongly support the "*Five Steps Forward for Food Allergy*" advocacy initiative announced yesterday by FAAN with the endorsement of nearly 70 organizations from across the country. These five steps include:

1.  passage of S. 1232, the Food Allergy and Anaphylaxis Management Act, to help schools create guidelines for managing food-allergic children;
2.  creation of a national clearinghouse at the Centers for Disease Control and Prevention on food allergy for the general public as well as health care professionals;
3.  development of national guidelines for the diagnosis and management of food allergy for health care professionals;
4.  significantly increased funding for research on food allergy and anaphylaxis; and
5.  expanded efforts by the U.S. Food and Drug Administration to improve food allergen labeling.

I would like to focus specific attention on the need for expanded research. In recent years, experts have been convened to identify the most promising avenues of research on food allergy and anaphylaxis:

*   In March of 2006, the NIH Expert Panel on Food Allergy, convened by the National Institute of Allergy and Infectious Disease (NIAID), released a report detailing an agenda of research questions that should be pursued if we are to succeed in identifying vaccines or improved treatments for food allergy. The report recommended additional basic and pre-clinical research on specific questions; clinical trials to evaluate promising new approaches to the prevention and treatment of food allergies; and expanded studies of the epidemiology and genetics of food allergy. The report also recommended that efforts be undertaken by the NIH and the FDA to resolve impediments to the design and conduct of clinical trials for the prevention and treatment of food allergy. Unfortunately, due to grossly inadequate funding, most of the research recommended in this report has not been pursued.

- In February of 2006, the Journal of Allergy and Clinical Immunology published the report of a symposium on anaphylaxis convened by the NIAID, the Academy, FAAN and others. This report detailed an agenda of research questions to be pursued to enable us to better understand anaphylaxis and improve methods for prevention and treatment. Again, due to grossly inadequate funding, most of these research initiatives have not been pursued.

Dr. Fauci is to be commended for the initiatives the NIAID has undertaken in the area of food allergy. I have been fortunate to be funded by the NIH for the past 25 years to support my research in food allergy. In that period of time, the field has moved from just trying to understand the manifestations of food allergy to the development of new diagnostic and treatment modalities, several of which are now just starting in clinical trials. However, I can tell you with absolute certainty that unless the Congress provides NIH with significant funding increases for research on food allergy and anaphylaxis, we will NOT make progress toward break-throughs in the prevention and treatment of food allergies. In addition, an investment must be made in the training of researchers in the field of allergy to pursue a significantly expanded research agenda in the areas of food allergy and anaphylaxis. FAAN is recommending annual increases of $10 million per year for five years (an additional $50 million over five years) to bring the budget for research on food allergy and anaphylaxis to a level that will allow us to pursue the research recommended in the two reports I have cited and to support the promising clinical trials underway. I strongly encourage this Committee to formally recognize this need and encourage the Appropriations Committee to provide this additional support at a minimum. I understand that the Federal budget is extremely tight at this time. However, it is important to recognize the size of this problem, over 10 million Americans and their families affected, and that most of the research necessary to improve methods of preventing and treating food allergy simply is not being done.

## CONCLUSION

Once again, I would like to thank you, Senator Dodd, for convening this important hearing. The American Academy of Allergy, Asthma and Immunology looks forward to working with you to achieve the enactment of S. 1232. In addition, we hope you and all members of this Committee will support the initiatives included in FAAN's "Five Steps Forward for Food Allergy" statement and that you will take steps to address the totally inadequate funding for research on food allergy.

Thank you for the opportunity to participate in this hearing. I would be happy to answer any questions.

In: Food Allergy Overview and Children's...    ISBN: 978-1-61728-478-6
Editor: Lee R. Daniels    © 2010 Nova Science Publishers, Inc.

*Chapter 9*

# STATEMENT OF DONNA KOSIOROWSKI, RN, MS, NCSN, ON BEHALF OF THE NATIONAL ASSOCIATION OF SCHOOL NURSES, HEARING ON "ADDRESSING THE CHALLENGE OF CHILDREN WITH FOOD ALLERGIES"[*]

## *Donna Kosiorowski*

Mr. Chairman, Mr. Alexander, and Members of the Subcommittee, I am Donna Kosiorowski, a practicing School Nurse Supervisor from West Haven, Connecticut School District, who is privileged to be here today representing the National Association of School Nurses (NASN) on the issue of addressing food allergies in schools. I commend the Subcommittee for bringing attention to the fact that more needs to be done to prepare our nation's schools to manage the risk of food allergy and anaphylaxis.

My testimony will explain that School Nurses are seeing increasing numbers of students with food allergies and the essential need to be prepared in the event a student has an anaphylactic reaction. I will also share with the Members of the Subcommittee personal experience with this issue over the

---

[*] This is an edited, reformatted and augmented version of a statement dated May 2008.

course of my 23 years in school nursing and offer Connecticut's response to these life threatening incidents in school as a model for other states.

NASN's membership of over 13,000 School Nurses are performing duties today that go well beyond what school nursing was like 30-40 years ago when health care costs were affordable and children with chronic health conditions were not "main-streamed." Even over the last 10 years, there have been rapid societal changes reflected in schools. Today, Federal laws like the Individuals with Disabilities Education Act (IDEA), result in children attending school in wheel chairs, on tube feedings, ventilators, central lines, pumps and other complex technologies. School Nurses are there to meet the needs of all students and the importance of managing life-threatening food allergies in the school setting is something that School Nurses are currently addressing. This life-threatening issue is recognized by NASN through the position statements we have included with our testimony and the informational resources we provide to our members.

School Nurses report an increase in the types of food allergies and other allergies in their school population. Approximately five to six percent of the general pediatric population have an incidence of food allergy, with eight foods (peanuts, shellfish, fish, tree nuts, eggs, milk, soy, and wheat) accounting for ninety percent of allergic reactions. However, children with food allergies can have good school attendance when a School Nurse is there to help them be healthy and safe at school. I think you will agree with the research that **Healthy Children Learn Better**. Knowing that healthy children learn better, School Nurses are working towards ensuring that all school districts will have the opportunity to consider adopting federal guidelines concerning the management of food allergies. Health needs and problems are not something children can leave at home. When they come to school, their health needs and problems come with them. They spend 6-8 hours per day at school. Data clearly demonstrate that fatalities associated with anaphylaxis occur more often away from home and are associated with the absence or delayed use of epinephrine. The School Nurse is a reliable and trusted health care provider and parents feel comfortable consulting with the School Nurse. It is the School Nurse who is often the child's first and only access into the health care system. We provide frontline care and if society wants children "not to be left behind," then nurses need to be there to help them stay healthy and in school so they can achieve academic success.

Now let me share with you Connecticut's 2006 law requiring the State Department of Education to develop guidelines for managing food allergies in school, which includes Food Allergy Management Plans. The Management

Plan is the basis for the development of guidelines implemented at the school level and provide for consistency across the state and in schools. The guidelines clearly outline prevention, education, awareness, communication and emergency response.

Consistency is important because all children must have standardized and appropriate individualized health care plans, developed through a formal process. This is protection for the children and families and consistency helps to prevent litigations. Plans should be based on medically accurate information and evidence-based practices using a process to identify, manage, and ensure continuity of care for students throughout their school career. Connecticut law allows School Nurses to train teachers, principals, coaches, and, in the case of epinephrine auto-injector, paraprofessionals, to administer medications to students with known allergies, not limited to food.

With or without guidelines for food allergy management, schools and school boards are obligated to maintain the health and protect the safety of any child with a health problem, including food allergies. Therefore, it is **necessary** for the United States Secretary of Health and Human Services to consult with the Secretary of Education on the development of a voluntary policy for managing the risk of food allergy and anaphylaxis in schools so that children are protected in a research-based and consistent manner. The federal mandates of IDEA and Section 504 of the Rehabilitation Act require schools that receive federal funding to provide certain medical services. In fortunate states, like Connecticut, who have a high ratio of school nurses-to-students, a plan of care is prepared and implemented by the school nurse. In a state like Tennessee, there are guidelines on the books, but the school nurse-to-student ratio is ranked 40th in the nation, which means that on average there is **1 nurse: 1,628 students**. Who will be there in those schools without nurses to implement the guidelines and ensure the safety of the children needing "rescue medication" like epinephrine? Having school-based food allergy management grants would greatly help local educational agencies throughout the country who are in need of **creating and *implementing*** guidelines, and hopefully as a result more school nurses will be placed in the schools to lead the effort.

Following are actual examples of how preparations for possible anaphylactic reactions make a difference in the lives of real school children:

Anaphylaxis has different symptoms in different people. Before Connecticut had their guidelines in place and they were implemented throughout the state, a girl with known food allergies, who I will call Sarah, came to the school nurse complaining of a stomach ache. Three times throughout the course of the day, the nurse sent her back to class. On her last trip back to the classroom, Sarah died from an anaphylactic reaction. This tragedy was clearly a result of not having a standard plan in place and a nurse who had not been properly trained to recognize all of the symptoms related to anaphylaxis. Lack of training plus no guidelines is a recipe for trouble.

On a positive note, when a family recently came to Connecticut from another state and wanted to register their little boy for kindergarten, the mother told the school nurse that her child, who I will call Danny, had severe food allergies and had been hospitalized several times for anaphylaxis. She further stated that the hospitalizations required intensive care and a tube to help him breathe. The mother claimed Danny had been denied entry to the school in the other state because there was no plan for "a child like him" and his health condition could not be managed safely in school. The previous school suggested consideration of home schooling. When coming to Connecticut, the mother was armed with information and knew the laws were on her side. The family was prepared to fight to get Danny into school with a plan to accommodate his special needs. Fortunately, the nurse was able to assure the mother that the Connecticut school district was ready and able to accommodate her child. Because Connecticut has strong guidelines, and nurses and other appropriate school staff have been trained for emergency situations, including established procedures with community EMS providers, Danny has remained safely in school.

Guidelines are a safeguard and protect both the child and the school district. Lack of guidelines can result in litigation and ultimately tragic deaths, as I described earlier. In Connecticut, I am aware of two court cases that were won by the school district because guidelines were implemented, individualized health care plans put in use, and staff training provided. Having a school district with every nurse trained to apply the same standard of care based on current guidelines is an ideal situation which has been honored by the courts. State guidelines give nurses a place to start and a process to follow which safeguards the student and the districts throughout the state. Although voluntary, the issuance of federal guidelines would greatly help support students who move from one state to another.

On behalf of the National Association of School Nurses, I implore this Subcommittee to move legislation that will provide a voluntary policy for managing the risk of food allergy and anaphylaxis in schools and will establish school-based food allergy management grants. With the growing number of students affected by food allergies, it is imperative that School Nurses have the support of the federal and state governments for the development of individualized health care plans, emergency plans, and procedures for safe medication administration and storage. Food allergies can be like a ghost hiding in the room. When they make their presence known, School Nurses want to stand fully prepared to make sure each and every child does not succumb to a preventable medical emergency.

# NATIONAL ASSOCIATION OF SCHOOL NURSES

## Position Statement

### The Role of School Nurses in AllergyAnaphylaxis Management

### History

Anaphylaxis can be deadly to children as well as adults. Among the general population, one to two percent are described as at risk for anaphylaxis from food and insects and a somewhat lower percentage are at risk from drugs and latex. Approximately five to six percent of the general pediatric population have an incidence of food allergy, with eight foods (peanuts, shellfish, fish, tree nuts, eggs, milk, soy, and wheat) accounting for 90% of allergic reactions. Food allergies are, in fact, the leading cause of anaphylaxis outside the hospital setting, accounting for an estimated 30,000 emergency room visits annually. It is estimated that 100 to 200 people die each year from food allergy-related reactions, and approximately 50 people die from insect sting reactions.

### Description of Issue

Care must be taken to differentiate between a true allergic response and an adverse reaction. True allergies result from an interaction between the allergen and the immune systems. Anaphylaxis is a potentially fatal reaction of multiple body systems. It can occur spontaneously. Data clearly demonstrate that fatalities associated with anaphylaxis occur more often away from home and are associated with the absence or delayed use of epinephrine.

### Rationale

Education and planning are key to establishing and maintaining a safe school environment for all students. Those responsible for the care and well being of children must be aware of the potential dangers of allergies. Prevention of allergy symptoms involves coordination and cooperation within the entire school team and should include parents, students, school nurses, and appropriate school personnel. Early recognition of symptoms and prompt interventions of appropriate therapy are vital to survival.

## Conclusion

It is the position of the National Association of School Nurses that schools have a basic duty to care for students, utilizing appropriate resources and personnel. School nurses are uniquely prepared to develop and implement individualized health care plans within state nurse practice act parameters and to coordinate the team approach required to manage students with the potential for experiencing allergic reactions.

## References/Resources

American Academy of Allergy, Asthma and Immunology Board of Directors (1998). Position Statement-Anaphylaxis in schools and other child-care settings. *Journal of Allergy Clinical Immunology, 102*(2), 173-175.

Food Allergy Network (2001). *Information about anaphylaxis: Commonly asked questions about anaphylaxis.* www.foodallergy.org.

Mudd, K. E. & Noone, S. A., (1995). Management of severe food allergy in the school setting. *Journal of School Nursing, 11*(3), 30-32.

National Association of School Nurses (2000). *Position Statement-Epinephrine use in life-threatening emergencies.* Scarborough, ME: Author.

Adopted:     November 2001

# NATIONAL ASSOCIATION OF SCHOOL NURSES

## Position Statement

### *Epinephrine Use in Life-Threatening Emergencies*

#### Summary

It is the position of the National Association of School Nurses that school nurses create and manage the implementation of emergency care plans for the treatment of life-threatening allergies in the school setting. State regulations, including nurse practice acts, will govern the need for protocols, standing orders, and/or individual orders for epinephrine administration.

## History

An increasing number of school students and staff have diagnosed life-threatening allergies, an abnormal immunologic response. Exposure to the affecting allergen can trigger anaphylaxis, an overwhelming systemic response, characterized by drop in blood pressure, respiratory distress, loss of consciousness, and potential death. Anaphylaxis requires emergent medical intervention with an injection of epinephrine but does not eliminate the need to call Emergency Medical Services (EMS). Epinephrine injection will stop the allergic response by opening the bronchiole airway passages for 10-20 minutes until more comprehensive emergency medical intervention can be obtained through the EMS system.

## Description of Issue

Avoidance of triggers, early recognition of symptoms, and immediate treatment are essential to the management of life-threatening allergies. There are both students and staff who have known life-threatening allergies, as well as those who have not been identified. Intervention with epinephrine is vital to saving lives.

Unfortunately, allergens of concern are readily encountered in the school environment and include food (5% children), insects (1% population), latex (1% population with increased incidence for those with spina bifida), medications, and exercise induced. Foods of primary concern are peanuts, tree nuts, fish, eggs, milk, wheat, and corn. Peanut allergy is rarely outgrown in adulthood. Allergy to cow's milk is more prevalent in children whereas shellfish allergy is more common in adults. Insects of concern are the species of Hymenoptera and include honeybees, wasps, yellow jackets, and hornets. Wasps and hornets are capable of stinging multiple times. Antibiotics are responsible for the majority of medication allergies and are less frequently present in the school setting (Mayo Clinic, Food Allergy).

## Rationale

Medication and emergency policies in school districts must be developed with the safety of all students and staff in mind. Easy access to and correct use of epinephrine are necessary to avoid life-threatening complications.

The school nurse, parent, health care provider, and student should evaluate the self-managed administration of epinephrine by a student on a case-by-case basis. Written permission from the parent and health care provider must be obtained for students with known life-threatening allergies who will self-medicate or who will have epinephrine administered by a school district employee. The decision to allow a student to self-carry and self-administer epinephrine should take into consideration the age/developmental level of the student, the school nurse's assessment of the student's ability to self medicate, the recommendations of the student's parent and health care provider, the need for a back-up supply, the specific school environment and the availability of a professional school nurse. The decision to delegate epinephrine administration to unlicensed assistive personnel is determined by state law and the professional nursing judgment of the school nurse (NASN, 2002).

An individual health care plan that includes periodic monitoring and nursing assessment, emergency plans, and evaluation should be written by the school nurse and maintained for every student with prescribed epinephrine. The school nurse should provide training for school staff in the recognition of life-threatening allergic reactions and the appropriate first aid/emergency measures that should be taken as determined by district policy and state law.

School districts must establish direction for handling episodes of anaphylaxis in students and staff with no previous history of life-threatening allergies. State laws governing nursing practice will determine the need for protocols, policies and procedures in the management of injectable epinephrine in the school setting.

## References/Resources

American Academy of Allergy, Asthma, and Immunology, 611 East Wells Street, Milwaukee, WI 53202. http://www.aaaai.org

Asthma and Allergy Foundation of America (AAFA), 1233 20th Street, NW, Suite 402, Washington, DC 20036. http://www.aafa.org

H.R. 2023 Asthmatic Schoolchildren's Treatment and Health Management Act of 2004.www.SchoolAsthma.com

Lieberman, P., Kemp, S. F., Oppenheimer, J., Lang, D.M., Bernstein, I. L., Niklas, R. A., et al. (2005). The diagnosis and management of anaphylaxis: An updated practice parameter. [Supp. 2] *The Journal of Allergy and Clinical Immunology, 115*(3).

Litarowsky, J. S., Murphy, S. O., & Canham, D. L. (2004). Evaluation of an anaphylaxis training program for unlicensed assistive personnel. *Journal of School Nursing, 20*(5), 279-284.

Mayo Clinic. *Food Allergy.* Retrieved April 2005 from http://www.mayoclinic.com/invoke.cfm?id=DS00082

National Association of School Nurses. (2002) *Position statement: Delegation.* Scarborough, ME: Author.

National Jewish Medical and Research Center. *http://www.nationaljewish.org* /diseaseinfo/diseases/allergy/index.aspx

Sicherer, S. H., Simons, F. E., (2004). Quandaries in prescribing an emergency action plan and self-injectable epinephrine for first-aid management of anaphylaxis in the community. *The Journal of Allergy and Clinical Immunology, 115*(3), 575-583.

Smit, D., Camerson, P. A, & Rainer, T. H. (2005) Anaphylaxis presentations to an emergency department in Hong Kong: Incidence and predictors of biphasic reactions. *Journal of Emergency Medicine, 28(4)*, 381-388.

Weiss, C., Munoz-Furlong, A., Ferlong, T. J., Arbit, J (2004). Impact of food allergies on school nursing practice. *Journal of School Nursing, 20(5)*, 268-278.

Adopted: Revised:
November 2000
June 2005

In: Food Allergy Overview and Children's...        ISBN: 978-1-61728-478-6
Editor: Lee R. Daniels                        © 2010 Nova Science Publishers, Inc.

*Chapter 10*

# STATEMENT OF COLENE BIRCHFIELD, MOTHER OF SON WITH SEVERE FOOD ALLERGIES, BEFORE THE SENATE HELP COMMITTEE, HEARING ON "ADDRESSING THE CHALLENGE OF CHILDREN WITH FOOD ALLERGIES"*

## *Colene Birchfield*

Good afternoon Chairman Dodd, Ranking Member Alexander and distinguished Members of the Committee. It is my privilege to appear before my home state Senator from Tennessee today. I deeply appreciate the opportunity to help the Committee gain a greater understanding of the personal difficulties that food allergic children and their families face every day. The number of children suffering from life-threatening food allergies is dramatically increasing nationwide, and I am thankful to the Committee for taking the time to address this alarming national children's health issue.

As an educator – I teach music education to elementary school children at Apison Elementary School in Ooltewah, Tennessee – I would also like to express my support for Senator Dodd's bill, S. 1232, and applaud the bill's

---

* This is an edited, reformatted and augmented version of a statement dated May 2008.

focus in providing our nation's schools with the necessary resources to protect children who suffer from life-threatening food allergies. Senator Dodd's bill, and the Committee's recognition of the importance of childhood food allergies, is encouraging, but there remains much to be done in the effort to prevent and cure food allergies.

When people hear the word "allergy," they may think of a runny nose or the sniffles. As I learned when my son Ryan was 3 months old, life-threatening food allergies are something very different than hay fever – and parents like me literally fear for our children's lives every day because an allergic individual's reaction to food can be so severe. Probably the scariest aspect of an allergic reaction to food is that each reaction can manifest in a different way. While one reaction might begin with a rapid succession of sneezing, another reaction may begin with lethargy, or hives. It's difficult enough for a parent to sometimes realize that their own child is having a reaction. Imagine a teacher who now needs to distinguish between the common cold and an allergic reaction. Our experience has been that many teachers just haven't been given the proper amount of education to understand how to identify a reaction and then how to treat one.

At 3 months old, Ryan was given milk formula and immediately began to vomit. Within minutes, he was covered head to toe in hives. Without hesitation, we took him to the emergency room. With Ryan being so young, and it being the height of flu season, the ER told us it was likely the flu and to just take him home and feed him like normal. Since I was mostly breast feeding at the time, it took probably another week before Ryan was fed another formula bottle. At that time, he reacted in the exact same way. We again rushed to the ER. This time, the doctor confirmed that a milk allergy was the likely culprit. Ryan needed to stay in the ER for several hours and be monitored to ensure a secondary reaction didn't occur. My husband and I were overwhelmed, as neither of our families had any members with food allergies. We spent the next several months educating ourselves as much as possible how to live with food allergies. We thought we had things covered, only to find out at about 10 months that Ryan was also allergic to egg. We had fed him a baby food jar that contained egg. This time, Ryan first swelled up around his mouth and broke out into hives. We recognized this reaction, even though it started a bit differently and immediately gave him the Benadryl. Thankfully, he had only had a bite and we were able to contain that reaction at home. It wasn't until a year old that Ryan was finally able to be formally tested for food allergies. The tests confirmed that he was severely allergic to both milk and egg. With Ryan now eating table food, we sprung into action to educate everyone around us. We carried cards that contained key words to identify the proteins for egg and milk that would help us with reading ingredients. Often times, we find that when people hear that a child has a food allergy, they only look for that main word (i.e.-milk or egg) to tell whether a food includes that allergen. What they don't realize is that an allergy to milk for example, means that the child cannot come into contact with any food containing any one of the 19 some odd milk proteins that exist. When reading labels, we must be diligent to look for all the variations of these protein words.

There is no "treatment" for life-threatening food allergies. Instead, children and their families must maintain a constant level of vigilance to avoid any kind of contact with the allergenic food. My child is allergic to milk, egg and peanut and avoiding these staples of the American food supply is a constant struggle. Here's an experiment you can try at home – go to your pantry and try to find even five foods that do not contain milk, egg or peanut. Now imagine that if you didn't read the label correctly, your child's life could be at risk. It is heart-wrenching from a parent's perspective to know that even with a high level of individual and parental responsibility, my child could still be endangered by a well-intentioned but uneducated teacher, caregiver, sports coach or even a server in a restaurant.

As you can imagine, mitigating risk for an infant is far simpler than when they enter the school system. When Ryan began preschool and then grade school, we were faced with a whole new world of complications for managing his medical condition. While some school systems have a broad program for handling medication, many individual schools have discretion to develop further, their own protocol for handling individual situations. My personal experience with schools is that the focus is primarily on peanut food allergies. While I am grateful that there is some awareness for the impact of a peanut allergy in a social/public situation, I think it's important for schools to understand that the potential for a life threatening reaction is also present for those with other food allergies. When registering my children for our current school, I was told that the school nurse is only in the building two days/week. This school's protocol is such that they lock medication in the nurse's office. All staff members are trained to use an epi-pen, of which we were thankful. The problem, as I explained to the staff, was that in the time it would take for a staff member to go to the nurse's office, unlock the medication, and bring it to him, Ryan could die. Often times, I get looked at and even remarks that I am being overly dramatic. They fail to realize that the rapid progression of anaphylactic reaction is a clearly documented medical emergency and should be treated as such. I insisted that Ryan needed to have the medication with him at all times. Time is of the essence in the event of any reaction. Going from a mild to a severe reaction can take seconds. I asked the school how they handle the lunchroom for children with allergies. This was the first year that our school has had a child with food allergies. There was another child enrolled who has a severe peanut allergy and the school accommodated him by allocating a "Peanut-Free" table. There is very limited space in the cafeteria, so this was the only exception made. I was told that Ryan could and should sit at the peanut-free table. While the school saw this as a safety precaution, I saw it as just as large a risk as if Ryan were integrated with all the other kids at any other table. The reason being, Ryan is allergic to more than just peanuts. He was now sitting at a table with a child who certainly wouldn't have peanuts, but did bring cheetos and egg products daily to the table and was sitting within inches of Ryan. This solution didn't help mitigate the risk for Ryan and it separated him from his own class. I will never feel entirely comfortable with the cafeteria situation, but I do know that I've educated the students in Ryan's class enough that they truly look out for him at lunch. Ryan now eats lunch with his class. He brings a "placemat" to put his food on, as the tables just get wiped off and not washed. Ryan's teacher delivers his medication to the lunchroom with Ryan each and every day.

As I said earlier, time is of the essence with any reaction. We learned this the very hard way. I share my story of Ryan's anaphylactic reaction to everyone who is willing to listen. We are his parents and we almost waited too long. Ryan had what one ER doctor we saw called a "perfect storm" reaction. He had contact with both milk and Bermuda grass, to which he is also allergic. Contact with these allergens caused an anaphylactic reaction. Ryan came in and just said he needed to sit down. He looked pale. We sat him down and he immediately started coughing. Now, Ryan had been playing outside, so we initially thought he could just be tired. Well, only seconds passed and we decided we better give him benadryl, as we thought he was starting to have a reaction. Within a couple of minutes, Ryan started sneezing uncontrollably and could hardly breather. We have a peak flow meter with which to test Ryan's breathing. When he is healthy, Ryan's peak flow is at 225. At the time of his reaction, he could barely hit 25. At this point, we decided we had to give Ryan the epinephrine. While my husband injected, I called 911. Epinephrine saved our son's life that day. We spent the night in the ER and came home more afraid than ever, but in a way, more empowered that we were able to handle the reaction.

The first thought that entered my mind when I came home was how fearful I am that if it took me, his mother, that long to react, how long will it take if the reaction happens at school? Do educators know enough to be able to handle such a life threatening situation in a timely manner? Do the kids know enough to tell that something is not right with Ryan?

Parents have to rely on everyone around their child to manage his food allergy. That's a scary scenario. Even simplicities such as playing on a playground are concerns for those with food allergies. While there isn't always food present on the playground, the risk is still present. Imagine a child who ate peanut butter and jelly and got peanut butter on their hands. They have not washed their hands and then go out to the playground. When the child who now has peanut residue touches the playground equipment, my child now becomes at risk. Ryan can react simply by touching something that contains the food residue to which he's allergic. Food allergy awareness and education needs to encompass the many different ways a child can be exposed. Many parents, myself included, with children who have severe food allergies carry wipes around and clean areas where their children play. We walk around perceived as being overly-protective, or perhaps even crazy, paranoid parents – just to try and reduce risk wherever possible. We're NOT crazy. We're scared. Allergen protein can be as life threatening to my child as a gun in the hands of a toddler.

Each and every day Ryan is placed in scenarios beyond his or our control. Children like Ryan are vulnerable to allergic reactions not only at school cafeterias and restaurants, but in any public setting, from childhood parties to an afternoon spent at a friend's house. Ryan has been invited to a sleepover at a classmate's home. I could not allow him to attend, because of his food allergies. There's just not enough understanding by the general public as to how serious this is. Ryan recently attended a birthday party where kids were jumping on a trampoline. The birthday boy had a bag of cheetos in his hand and decided to jump on the trampoline with them. Ryan immediately told the boy he couldn't be around him if the child was going to have cheetos on his hand, as it could hurt him. Ryan proceeded to get off the trampoline and would not go back on. Seems like such a simple thing to most people. To me, that was a huge victory. I've educated Ryan enough that he is able to stand up for his own safety. I can only hope and pray that this will continue. As children grow up, they are going to test boundaries and push limits – a natural part of the maturation process. With the food allergic child, the teenage years can be particularly frightening as the kids struggle to fit in and "prove" their normalcy. One of my greatest fears is that my son will play down or try to hide his allergy from his peers out of a desire to not want to be "different." If the people around him do not understand his allergies, they cannot help him in an emergency situation.

Efforts to protect our children in school, and other social settings are very important. However, what we need more than anything else is research to find a cure for life-threatening food allergies. Ryan participated in an exciting research study based at Duke University Medical Center in North Carolina. On each visit, Ryan was given small amounts of milk protein, exposing him to the very thing to which he is deathly allergic. The first visit caused an anaphylactic reaction that came on with rapid speed. The doctors and nurses were very well prepared, as they expected this type of reaction. I was asked by a friend who has a child with a peanut allergy how I could sit there and purposely cause my son to have that reaction. Well, my answer is simple. How could I not afford him the opportunity for a lifetime without the risk of this type of reaction occurring again? The hope was that, over time, he would build up a sort of immunity – they call it desensitization – and would be able to tolerate milk later in his life. Our participation in the Duke study is a good example of just how desperate parents of food allergic children are to find any kind of relief for our children. We drove 7 ½ hours each way to get to Duke because there are no facilities that we know of closer to home that are doing this kind of work. We stayed in town near Duke when we would have to make the visits and there was a constant danger that my son would have a severe, adverse reaction to the treatment. In fact, numerous times, Ryan had little mini reactions, like hives on his back or a few coughs. The doctors are, after all, feeding him something that could kill him.

Why are we willing to subject our son to this risk? Because he faces a greater risk every single day of his life simply by being surrounded by foods that can harm him. Research is our only hope for a long-term solution to these deadly allergies. There's no distance I wouldn't travel for the possibility of alleviating the daily risk Ryan faces. You know, the old saying "No Risk, No Reward" is how I feel about the research. There's never a guarantee that these research studies are going to "cure" my child. To not participate is almost guaranteeing the status quo – enrolling in the study offers hope. At the very least, we've contributed to the research. At best, we may have found a way to live without fear that our child could die from food.

You can help us. Millions of parents just like me are counting on the US Congress to increase the amount of research that is conducted on life-threatening food allergies. There are only a handful of research centers like Duke around the county that are currently doing any kind of food allergy research. After 11 months of participation in Duke's Research Study, Ryan is now able to tolerate milk. This is a huge victory for both Ryan and the study itself. Ryan can now come into contact with any milk protein and not have to reach for the epi-pen. The study has proven to work in his case. There is still much more research to be done. For example, we know that as long as Ryan has a daily dose of milk protein, he's ok. What we don't know is what happens if he goes without for days on end. This is where the research still needs to continue. We are a unique glimpse at what can be accomplished. The federal government currently spends under $10 million a year funding research on food allergies. That is simply not enough. We need new research studies, more researchers and doctors investigating the disease, and funding to allow the best scientific minds in the field to find a cure.

Like any parent, I simply want my child to have the opportunity to grow and flourish in his life, and to reach his potential without limitations. On behalf of Ryan and the millions of other kids just like him, I am begging for your help.

Thank you!

# INDEX

**F**

**G**

**H**